June, 2009   Beijing

# Chinese Acupressure Therapy

Wang Zhaopu

FOREIGN LANGUAGES PRESS   BEIJING

First Edition 1999

Home Page:
http://www.flp.com.cn
E-mail Addresses:
info@flp.com.cn
sales@flp.com.cn

ISBN 7-119-02056-0

© Foreign Languages Press, 1999
Published by Foreign Languages Press
24 Baiwanzhuang Road, Beijing 100037, China

Printed by Beijing Foreign Languages Printing House
19 Chegongzhuang Xilu, Beijing 100044, China

Distributed by China International Book Trading Corporation
35 Chegongzhuang Xilu, Beijing 100044, China
P.O. Box 399, Beijing, China

*Printed in the People's Republic of China*

# Contents

# *Preface*

One of the most deadly movements in Chinese martial arts is *Dianxue*, i.e., striking with the finger at a selected point on the opponent's body, so as to incapacitate him at once for at least a short while. For 2,000 years, Chinese martial artists have used this skill to subdue rivals. However, it was not until the founding of the People's Republic that the method was refined by traditional doctors to treat both common diseases and complicated ones such as cerebral palsy and poliomyelitis. This remedial form of treatment came to be known as acupressure therapy.

While acupuncture and moxibustion are widely known and practised, acupressure therapy has until recently received little attention amongst the general public. The therapy involves percussing, pressing and massaging selected acupoints and stimulation-lines on the body's surface with the fingers.

In the last seven years or so, the Bone Disease Department of the Institute of Orthopaedics and Traumatology under the China Academy of Traditional Chinese Medicine has studied and applied this therapy with satisfactory results. A good collection of clinical data and scientific topical research based on modern technology have advanced the modernization of traditional Chinese medicine in this particular field.

Chinese acupressure therapy has already attracted the attention of medical workers in other countries. They have either come to China to study it, or referred their patients to acupressure specialists in China. Meanwhile, Chinese specialists have been invited to other countries to give lectures and demonstrations. The growing interest in this therapy outside of China has prompted me to write this book for the benefit of our counterparts abroad.

This book consists of three chapters. The first chapter includes a general introduction, a brief history of the therapy, points of attention in clinical application, modes of manipulation, indications and contraindications, and a list of acupoints and stimulation-lines. The second chapter deals with the clinical application of the therapy in treating diseases of the nervous system and the system of bones and joints, and some common syndromes. It also includes case reports. The third chapter dwells on clinical and laboratory research, including a number of case reports on the sequelae of cerebral birth injury, cerebral trauma and injury of the spinal column. The lab research includes topics on somatosensory evoked potential, electromyography, immunology, cardiovascular function, microcirculation of the fingernail fold, measurement of regional cerebral blood flow and microcirculation of the cerebral cortex, hemorrheology in experimental animals and the influence of acupressure manipulation on the neuron-transmitter in blood. These studies reveal that the mechanism of the therapy improves the patient's blood circulation and his organic metabolism, thereby ameliorating the function of the diseased parts. They demonstrate the soundness of the traditional Chinese medical (TCM) theory of "activating blood circulation and expelling hemostagnation" in the clinical application of acupressure therapy.

We sincerely look forward to comments from the readers, which will help us improve the book in the next edition.

Professor Wang Zhaopu
1991

# Chapter One
## General Introduction

### *Section I*
### Origin of Acupressure Therapy and Its Current Status

Acupressure therapy has evolved from the traditional Chinese martial art of *Dianxue* which is the technique of hitting hard at a selected acupoint on the opponent's body so as to momentarily block the flow of blood and energy and cause unconsciousness. Based on the same theory, the acupressure therapist skilfully fingers the same acupoint to promote the flow of blood and energy and heal an injury.

Chinese martial arts, particularly the art of *Dianxue*, has traditionally been shrouded in mystery in countless legendary tales from early centuries. Authentic historical records of this art are rare and fragmentary. One of the earliest remains that bear witness to this ancient tradition to this day, is the Shaolin Temple, deep in the Songshan Mountains thirteen kilometres northwest of present-day Dengfeng County, in Henan Province, central China. Chinese official dynastic history shows that in A.D. 495, the Northern Wei Emperor Xiaowen decreed the building of this temple for the revered Indian Buddhist Bhadra, who had come to China to spread his religion. In A.D. 527, another Indian Buddhist, Bodhidharma, came to this temple to preach. As his disciples sat long hours in meditation, they needed exercise to stretch their muscles. Besides, prowling wild beasts in the surrounding mountains created the need for martial art skills for self-defence.

Bodhidharma designed a series of eighteen body movements after the fashion of a leaping tiger, a climbing monkey, a flying bird, a crawling snake and so on, incorporating them into two martial art classics—the "Xisui" (washing of marrow) and the "Yijin" (change of tendons). The former has been lost in antiquity; the latter, which was deposited in the Shaolin Temple, was practised and refined through the centuries before it finally developed into what is now known as the Shaolin school of martial arts.

The technique of *Dianxue* originated from the fabulous martial artist Zhang Sanfeng, a Taoist priest from northeast China. The *Book of Ming History* records that two Ming emperors, Taizu (1368-1398) and Chengzu (1403-1424), had both tried, in vain, to seek him out in the mountains. In his later years, Zhang discovered seventy-two acupoints on the body vulnerable to *Dianxue*.

Throughout centuries of continuous refinement, the Shaolin martial art became a formidable weaponless fighting technique, so much so that in A.D. 1553, when a contingent of Japanese pillaging warriors, vagrants and traders set foot on Chinese soil, the Chinese resistance comprised martial-art monks originating from the Shaolin Temple.

Concomitant with the perfection of the Shaolin martial arts, there arose the need for remedies for injuries caused by it. In the Ming and Qing dynasties (1368-1911) a therapeutic system which took on the name of "Shaolin traumatology" developed into a branch of traditional Chinese medicine specializing in the treatment of injuries of bones, sinews and muscles. A school of traumatologists within this system began using the theories of the devastative technique of *Dianxue* to serve a therapeutic purpose, thus marking the inception of present-day acupressure therapy.

As the power of the *Dianxue* technique is determined by pinpointing the right acupoint with energized fingers, the success of acupressure likewise depends on the correct manipulation by the fingers, the correct selection of acupoints and the art of energizing the fingertips. The seventy-two acupoints listed by Zhang Sanfeng more than 500 years ago are still among those used by acupressure therapists today.

In 1950, a year after the founding of the People's Republic, an institution using nerve stimulation as a therapy was established in Beijing. Research work followed under the guidance of the Chinese Academy of Traditional Chinese Medicine to study the diagnostic value of acupressure and the theory of stimulation-lines in the body. In the ensuing years, a number of books and papers based on successful clinical experience and lab research were published. Since 1965, application of this therapy has been extended from traumatic inflictions to certain refractory diseases with satisfactory results. In the late seventies, the author of this book, together with doctors and researchers of the Institute of Orthopedics and Traumatology under the Chinese Academy of TCM, had proved the efficacy of this therapy in a number of other diseases. In 1983, acupressure treatment of sequelae of cerebral damage during delivery was for the first time taken up by the author and his colleagues in the Institute as a topic for clinical and lab research. The results were positive, and were published in two major monographs in 1985 and 1987.*

Training classes for acupressure therapy have been organized by the Institute of Orthopedics and Traumatology under the Chinese Academy of TCM. Some 150 practitioners from Beijing, Shanghai and Shandong Province have received training and begun practising the therapy with satisfactory results. Dr. Jia Lihui, an acupressure specialist, has trained many more practitioners in this therapy, in Shandong and some other provinces.

The author has given many well-received lectures on acupressure therapy in Tokyo, Yokohama and Hiroshima in Japan, and more recently, in Australia. Doctors and medical delegations from the United States, France, Japan, Switzerland and the Philippines have come to China to share ideas and experience in this particular field. The academic papers from China presented at two international symposiums on the treatment of cerebral paralysis and taut-foot by acupressure therapy, have been well received.

---

*"Acupressure treatment of sequelae of old injuries of the cerebrum and cervical spinal cord associated with functional disturbance of extremities and trunk" (1985); "Study on the mechanism and effect of acupressure therapy on 300 cases of sequelae of cerebral damage during delivery" (1987).

Efforts to research and perfect this therapy, in addition to the publicity it has so far received both at home and abroad, fall far short of the attention it really deserves, and its practitioners are still relatively few. Obviously the field is wide open for further advances in this therapeutic method, both in China and other countries.

## Section II
# What Is Acupressure?

Acupressure therapy, a legacy of traditional Chinese medicine, is administered by percussing and/or pressing with the fingers on the selected acupoints and stimulation-lines underneath the skin, so as to restore the functions of incapacitated parts of the body. Evolved from the Chinese martial arts (*wushu*), its methodology modifies the powerful karate movements to make them amenable to the human body. The mode of application varies with the characteristics of the affliction, but is on the whole simple and requires no drugs or instruments. It is safe, easy to learn, practicable almost anywhere and therefore suitable for popularization.

## Section III
# General and Local Effects of Acupressure Therapy

## A. General Effects

1. General relaxation, sound sleep, good appetite, increase of body weight and strength. Body temperature may rise 1-3°C after one manipulation.
The therapy increases the body's natural immunity against diseases.
2. Improvement of cardiovascular function. The therapy lowers arterial diastolic pressure and increases pulse pressure. It may also lower the peripheral resistance of arterioles, especially that of the microcirculatory system, thus improving the general cardiovascular function.
3. Improvement of microcirculatory function. After a single manipulation, micro-circulation of the fingernail fold improves and blood circulation accelerates; the calibre of the capillary loop widens and becomes better filled; and corpuscle congregation disappears, indicating the improvement of peripheral circulation.
4. Improvement of cerebral microcirculation. The volume of blood flowing into the brain increases, thus improving the supply of oxygen and nutrients and stimulating the discharge of metabolites, which facilitates the recovery of the cerebrum.
5. The conductive function of the nervous system improves, thus increasing sensitivity towards external stimuli.
6. It decreases the amount of noradrenaline and dopamine, thus improving blood circulation.
7. It activates blood circulation and dissipates blood stagnation by removing excessive viscosity, concentration, coagulation and congregation of the blood.
8. For the digestive system, the therapy relieves enteric spasm, dyspepsia and diarrhoea in children, as well as other diseases of the digestive tract.
9. The most convincing example of its therapeutic value to the excretory system

is its effectiveness in curing all kinds of enuresis.

In short, through research and clinical application, acupressure therapy has been proved effective on many parts of the body. Further research on the subject is expected to result in fresh discoveries and new scientific interpretations.

### B. Local Effects

The manipulated locality feels sore, numb, dilated and painful. The skin turns red, and the swelling and muscle spasm disappears. Mild stimulation is analgesic while strong stimulation causes pain, with local sweating and a rise in skin temperature.

## Section IV
# Therapeutic Actions of Acupressure Therapy

### A. Regulation of *Yin* and *Yang*

According to the concept of traditional Chinese medicine, everything in the universe is made up of two forces, *Yin* and *Yang*, opposing and supplementing each other. When *Yin* and *Yang* are in harmony, health is ensured; when the two are in disharmony, there is illness. The same holds true regarding the human body. Flexion of the joints and adduction of the limbs are categorized under *Yin*, whilst straightening of the joints and abduction of the limbs are classified under *Yang*. In patients with sequelae of cerebral injury resulting in muscle spasm causing digital and elbow flexion, foot and wrist ptosis, and adduction of the thighs, the syndrome indicates a preponderance of *Yin* and deficiency of *Yang*.

Treatment with acupressure therapy involves strong stimulation of the points on the stimulation-lines along the medial (*Yin*) aspects of the upper and lower limbs by means of percussing and pressing these points to reduce excessive *Yin*, whilst moderate manipulation of the points along the stimulation-lines on the lateral (*Yang*) aspects of the limbs, supplemented by mildly poking the toes, will relieve the spasm. Amelioration or total cure of the ailment is the result of the re-regulation of *Yin* and *Yang*, which restores the reflexes in the joints and the functions of the hands, feet and limbs. Examination of somatosensory evoked potential reveals a normal or nearly normal latent period, which coincides with the improved physical signs. This to some extent reflects the soundness of the *Yin/Yang* thesis.

### B. Dredging the Meridians

In the case of body injury, there is usually stagnation of blood and vital energy at the injured spot resulting in numbness, swelling, stiffness, pain or even visceral disorder. This is especially common with the sequelae of old brain or cervical spinal injuries, particularly in cases of cerebral paralysis. Acupressure therapy removes obstruction in the flow of vital energy by pressing the meridians, and dissipates the blockage by massaging the swollen area. Thus the resilience of muscles and tendons is recovered and the spasm is remitted or stopped altogether. Foot ptosis, scissor legs, adducted thumb and flexed elbow can be cured, and functional disturbances caused by partial injury of neurons (peripheral nerves) can be overcome in this way. Laboratory diagnosis shows that after acupressure therapy, the pathological waves disappear from the electromyographs of these patients, and the latent period of somatosensory evoked potential returns to normal. This explains the theory of dredging the meridians.

## C. Co-ordinating the Flow of *Qi*

Lu Shidao, an ancient Chinese doctor said: "When the body is injured by external factors, the flow of vital energy and blood will be injured internally, resulting in the blockage of defensive and nutrient energies and disharmony of the viscera." It is essential that the blood and vital energy should move and circulate. In case they become stagnant, manifestations such as muscular spasm, dry skin, cold and cyanotic fingers and toes, edema, swelling, soreness, pain and numbness would ensue. Acupressure therapy restores the flow of vital energy and blood. Thus the viscera are regulated, the limbs strengthened, the atrophic muscles restored to normal, swelling and edema dissipated, pain and numbness relieved or subdued, and the movement of the joints restored. Laboratory examination reveals that the improvement of cardiovascular functions is mainly due to a decrease in peripheral resistance of the blood vessels and diastolic pressure, and an increase in the systolic pressure rate and velocity of capillary blood flow. All this results in the improvement of microcirculation in the patient which, according to the concept of traditional Chinese medicine, indicates proper co-ordination of the *qi* and blood.

## D. Lysis of Adhesion

Acupressure therapy, supplemented with orthopedic manipulation, is good for relieving adhesion of the joints at the shoulder, elbow, hip, knee, ankle, finger and toe. The manipulative movements should be mild at the beginning. Extend or flex the joints and simultaneously manipulate them to gradually increase their range of movement. Abrupt movements should be avoided or the ligaments and synovial sac would be injured, or fractures might even occur.

## E. Relieving Muscle Spasm and Increasing Muscle Strength

Clinically, it can be demonstrated that acupressure therapy is effective in curing not only muscle spasm in cerebral palsy but also muscle atrophy in sequelae of infantile paralysis. For muscle spasm, manipulation is heavy, whereas for flaccid muscular paralysis, mild manipulation is applied.

## F. Strengthening Resistance and Dispelling and Attacking
## Pathogenic Factors

Cellular immunity was examined in 27 cases, aged 1-10, of sequelae of cerebral birth injury. After treatment with acupressure, local skin temperature increased by 1-3°C, the manipulated area reddened and the patient felt comfortable and relaxed. Other manifestations included sound sleep, good appetite, increase of body strength and less susceptibility to common cold. The therapy obviously not only acts upon the nervous and cardiovascular systems but improves the immunity of the body. The results definitely demonstrate that acupressure therapy is capable of strengthening body resistance, harmonizing vital energy and blood circulation and dredging the meridians.

*Section V*

# Indications and Contraindications of Acupressure Therapy

## A. Indications

1. Diseases of the nervous system: Sequelae of cerebral birth injury and brain diseases, trauma, partial paralysis caused by injury of the spinal column, sequelae of poliomyelitis, multiple neuritis, arachnoidal adhesion, cerebral paralysis, facial paralysis, partial paralysis of plexus brachialis nerve, partial injury of nervous medians, nervus ulnaris, nervus radialis, sciatic nerve and nervus peroneus communis.

2. Diseases of the spine: Cervical vertebral syndromes, stiff neck, torticollis, disorder of posterior lumbar joints, herniation of the third lumbar bone syndromes, herniation of the lumbar intervertebral disc, derangement of intervertebral articulation.

3. Diseases of the joints of the arms and legs.

4. Other symptoms: headache, toothache, hiccup, infantile indigestion, common cold, bed-wetting, hypochondriasis, drooling, foot and wrist ptosis.

## B. Contraindications

The following conditions should not be treated with acupressure therapy.

1. Acute diseases, infectious diseases, acute stomachache, suppurative arthritis.
2. Severe heart diseases, tuberculosis, malignant tumors.
3. Hemorrhagic diseases such as hemophilia and purpura.
4. Severe skin diseases.

*Section VI*

# Preparations Prior to Treatment

Prior to treatment, besides preparing the case history, making necessary physical and laboratory examinations and giving a correct diagnosis, the doctor should indicate to the patient the relatively long process of treatment and the prospects for recovery so as to enhance his understanding, patience and confidence and win his co-operation in the course of treatment.

The clinic room should be spacious, well ventilated and illuminated. The examination table should be adjusted to an appropriate height. Necessary instruments including stethoscope, angle square, percussion hammer, tape measure, otoscope, ophthalmoscope, sphygmomanometre, tuning fork, and electric torch should be laid out.

The manipulators should frequently trim finger nails but without overdoing it, so as not to hurt the finger-tips or nail grooves, which can be protected by adhesive plaster if necessary.

## *Section VII*

# Points of Attention in Clinical Practice

1. On the basis of case history and lab reports such as EMGs, cardiograms, somatosensory evoked potential charts, make an overall analysis of the illness and the patient's condition before deciding on the acupoints and stimulation-lines for each individual patient. This is especially important in the following cases: debilitated children, starving or overfed people, patients on their first visit and women during menstruation. The therapy should not be practised on patients under the influence of liquor or in a state of physical exhaustion. Deformities should be treated with great patience.

2. Start the manipulations lightly, gradually increase in intensity and wind up with light movements. Special care should be taken to avoid injuring joint capsules, tendons and bones.

3. The patients usually have such sensations as soreness, numbness, warmth, spasm and distension in the area of manipulation. Skin flush may occur; sometimes the patients may sweat or experience fever. Subcutaneous bleeding may occur in the beginning, but will gradually disappear in a week. None of these reactions require any special treatment.

In case of severe reactions such as dizziness, nausea, vomiting, loss of colour or shock, the manipulation should be stopped and relaxation techniques applied immediately, such as clapping the patient on the head, back or shoulders, pressing Bige and Yongquan (KI 1), poking the finger and toe radixes quickly, and massaging the trigonum lumbale and abdominal walls.

With some patients, symptoms may be aggravated after initial treatment with acupressure therapy, but the aggravation will finally disappear in three to five days.

4. Frequency and duration of treatment. The manipulation is usually performed once a day or every other day, depending on the reaction of the patient. For mild cases, a course of treatment usually lasts ten days; for chronic cases, it lasts one to two months.

If the curative effect is slow, it is advisable to discontinue treatment for two or three weeks before it is resumed.

## *Section VIII*

# Learning the Acupressure Technique

The beginner should initially acquire a general knowledge of human anatomy and body functions. He should be familiar with the system of acupoints and train in manipulating the hands and fingers. It is recommended that he should begin by letting his teacher locate the acupoints on his own body and manipulate them so as to feel for himself the sensation this creates. Since an acupressure manipulator requires strength and physical stamina, he should take plenty of exercise, paying special attention to his arms, wrists and fingers so as to keep them strong and flexible, in order that he can use them whenever the occasion requires, so as to achieve optimum results. Thus the beginner is advised to train in the following steps:

1. To practise manipulating the hands and fingers until he is familiar with the different modes of application.

2. To familiarize himself with the positions of his own acupoints and stimulation-lines, and feel for himself their varying reactions to self-administered acupressure manipulation. This will help him to locate the proper acupoints and apply acupressure to an appropriate degree in clinical practice.

3. To sum up clinical experience from time to time for the benefit both of himself and others.

## Section IX
# Acupressure Techniques

Acupressure involves five basic manipulation techniques and twelve auxiliary ones. Clinical application usually combines both techniques.

### A. The Five Basic Manipulations

1. Percussion. This is the major manipulation technique applicable to both the acupoints and the stimulation-lines. There are three varieties:

a. One-finger percussion, mainly using the middle finger. Slightly flex the palm and the phalanges, with the index finger doubled up with the middle finger, the finger pad of the thumb pressed against the distal phalange of the middle finger, and the ring and little fingers clenched. This technique is used mainly for heavy percussion. (See Fig. 1)

b. Three-finger percussion, using the index and middle fingers and the thumb. Slightly flex the palm with the thumb pressed against the finger balls of the index and middle fingers, and the ring and little fingers clenched. (See Fig. 2)

c. Five-finger percussion, with the fingers slightly flexed and the finger tips adducted. (See Fig. 3)

The manipulator percusses by co-ordinating the movements of the shoulder, elbow and wrist. Whilst focusing his attention upon the manipulation, he consciously directs his strength and energy to the tips of the fingers, holding them at an angle of 60°-90°

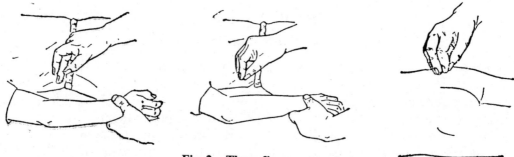

Fig. 2    Three-finger percussion

Fig. 1    One-finger percussion

Fig. 3    Five-finger percussion

to the body. He then starts to percuss at an average pace of 2-3 times per second. The percussion movements are usually rhythmical in four different patterns: 1 weak and 2 strong, 2 weak and 2 strong, 3 weak and 2 strong, and 5 weak and 2 strong. The strong percussions are slightly slower than the weak ones, but should be snappy, solid, yet tender at the same time.

The percussion movement falls into three categories in terms of strength.

a. Light percussion, mainly using the wrist, supported by the elbow and shoulder joints. This method offers light stimulation as an auxiliary remedy. It is usually applied to children, women, old and weak patients, and patients indicating deficiency of vital energy and lowered body resistance.

b. Medium percussion, mainly using the elbow and the forearm with the wrist joint in a fixed or semifixed position. The shoulder joint plays a supportive role. This is used for patients who show either deficiency or excessive syndromes.

c. Strong percussion, mainly using the shoulder joint and the upper arm, with the wrist joint fixed and the elbow joint in a co-ordinating position. This is applied to stronger patients and young adults, or when the painful point is located under thick soft tissue or deep under the skin. Usually, strong percussion is applied to cases with excessive symptom-complex.

*Training methods.*

Generally the training proceeds from light to medium and then to strong percussion, with emphasis on practising the use of the wrist, elbow and shoulder joints and regulating the pace and accuracy of the percussion movements.

(1) Practice on sandbag. Make a round sandbag of about $10 \times 10$ cm in diameter and 3 cm in thickness, and draw a small circle about the size of the finger tip in the centre. Hold the sandbag with one hand and do the one-, three- and five-finger percussion on the mark, paying particular attention to precision. For beginners, the percussion movements need not be strong. Increase the force of the percussion gradually as the trainee familiarizes himself with the movements. Never practise on a hard surface to avoid hurting the finger-tips.

(2) Practice on your own body. This may follow the practice on the sandbag so as to have personal experience of the percussion sensation. Percuss along the stimulation-lines, and when an acupoint is reached, percuss with heavier force.

2. Pressing. Done with the thumb, this is one of the most commonly used manipulation techniques. The four fingers are either spread on one side of the afflicted area to support the thumb, or clenched with the index finger kept close to the thumb. (See Figs. 4 & 5) Press the tip of the thumb on the selected point and move forward, backward, right, left and then in a circle, but never lift the thumb from the skin. The tip of the thumb is kept at a 45°-90° angle to the skin. The pressing technique, applied mostly in the case of excessive syndrome, produces strong stimulation to relieve pain and spasm or serve a sedative purpose.

3. Poking with fingernail. The manipulator uses the nail of his thumb or index finger to poke at the selected points on the nail radixes and phalangeal joints of the patient's fingers or toes. He holds his patient's wrist or ankle with one hand to keep it in a fixed position, and perform the manipulation with the other hand, slightly lifting

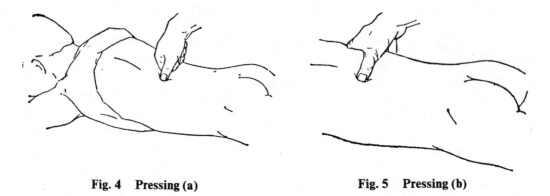

Fig. 4    Pressing (a)                  Fig. 5    Pressing (b)

the finger or toe to facilitate manipulation. The intensity of the poking varies with the condition and age of the patient. Start with light poking and increase intensity as required. Indications: Paralysis of lower extremities, headache, common cold. (See Fig. 6)

4. Clapping. The manipulator adducts and slightly flexes his fingers and puts the finger pad of the thumb close to the index finger so that when he claps with the hand, only the finger pads, the thenar and the hypothenar touch the skin. (See Fig. 7)

This technique produces medium stimulation. It mainly uses the force of the elbow, with the wrist in a fixed position or moving slightly, and the shoulder muscles co-ordinating with the clapping movement. When clapping the chest area, the patient should be told to draw a deep breath thoracically and hold it while the clapping goes on. Clap lightly 5-10 times at the start. Gradually increase the number of times and the force of the strokes, depending on the patient's physical conditions. When clapping the abdominal area, the patient should breathe abdominally. The therapist should take care not to damage the intestines.

The clapping technique promotes the normal flow of blood and vital energy which serves to relax muscles and tendons, strengthen the spleen, stomach and kidney, improve general health and relieve such symptoms as respiratory distress and dizziness caused by excessive acupressure manipulations. It is usually applied on the head and back and sometimes on the abdomen to treat enuresis.

5. Knocking.

a. Knocking with the finger-tips adducted and the fingers slightly flexed, the tip of the thumb touching the radial side of the index finger. The knocking provides strong stimulation. The method of application and the functions are the same as for percussion. (See Fig. 8)

b. Knocking with the palm side of the five fingers, using the same technique as clapping. This provides a milder stimulation and is applied to the head or other parts of the body to relax muscular spasm or pain in the area of acupressure therapy.

## B. Supplementary Manipulations

### 1. Orthopaedic manipulations

Orthopaedic manipulation is a necessary supplement to acupressure in dealing

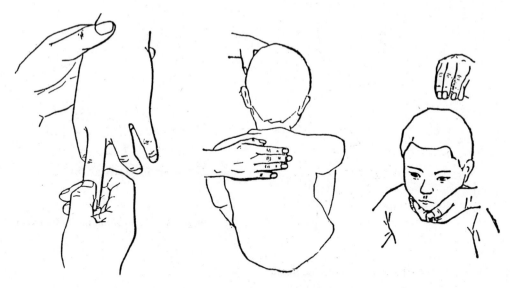

**Fig. 6   Poking with fingernail**      **Fig. 7   Clapping**      **Fig. 8   Knocking**

with deformities of the extremities.

1. Orthopaedic manipulation of the shoulder joint. Let the patient:

a. Raise the arm to 180°, if possible. The patient may need help from the doctor. (See Fig. 9)

b. Wipe the frontal region with the upper portion of the forearm. Elbow bends at 90°. (See Fig. 10)

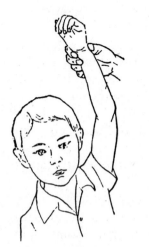
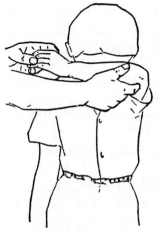
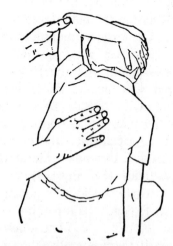

**Fig. 9   Raise the arm**      **Fig. 10   Rub forehead with upper portion of the forearm**      **Fig. 11   Touch the opposite auricle with the fingers from behind the head**

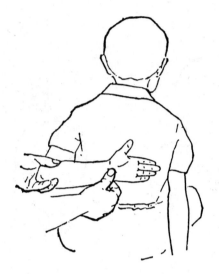

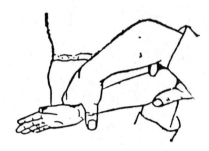

Fig. 13    **Supination of the forearm**

Fig. 12    **Touch the spine with the thumb**

c. Touch the opposite auricle with the fingers from behind the head. (See Fig. 11)

d. Touch the spine with the thumb. (See Fig. 12)

If the patient has difficulties with these exercises, acupressure methods such as percussion, pressing or massage may be applied to help relax the contracted muscles. The combination of orthopaedic and acupressure manipulations facilitates both diagnostic and clinical treatment.

2. Orthopaedic manipulation of the forearm.

When there is disturbance to the supination of the forearm, flex the elbow joint to 90°. The doctor holds the patient's posterior portion of the elbow joint with one hand and the lower portion of the forearm with the other hand. Rotate the forearm and hand so that the palm faces upward. Repeat 20-30 times. (See Fig. 13)

3. Orthopaedic manipulation of the wrist and hand

To correct ptosis of the wrist and hand, the doctor puts both thumbs on the patient's palm and the fingers of both hands on the dorsal region of the wrist. Knead with the thumbs in the direction of the thenar and the hypothenar to relax spasm of the muscles of the palm. Continue to knead from the bases of the thumb and the index, middle, ring, and little fingers to their tips, to correct their contraction. Meanwhile, the doctor adducts his fingers and presses the wrist's dorsal region with the ulnar side of the little fingers to correct ptosis of the wrist. Repeat 20-30 times. (See Fig. 14)

4. Orthopaedic manipulation of the hip joint

a. Expand the hip joint. The patient lies in a supine position and flexes both knee joints to 90°. The doctor holds the medial sides of both knee joints and separates them laterally, then massages along the gracilis, the adductor magnus, the adductor longus and the sartorius to correct adductive contraction of the hip joint.

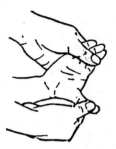

**Fig. 14   Orthopaedic manipulation of wrist and hand**

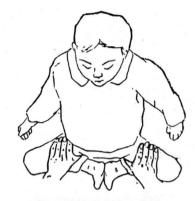

**Fig. 15   Expanding the hip joint**

(See Fig. 15)

b. Stretch and elevate the leg and massage along the posterior aspect of the thigh with three fingers. The patient lies in a supine position and extends the afflicted leg. The doctor lifts it with his left hand, resting the patient's knee against his left elbow and raising the leg as far as it can go. Meanwhile the doctor adducts his right index, middle and ring fingers and massages the upper portion of the patient's posterior aspect of the thigh along the contracted semitendinosus and semimembranosus and the biceps femoris downward to the insertions. At the same time elevate the extended leg continuously until it reaches the normal range. Repeat 20-30 times. (See Fig. 16)

c. Medial rotation of the hip joint at the head and neck of the femur. The patient lies in a supine position and flexes both the hip and knee joints to 90°. The doctor holds the anterior portion of the knee joint with one hand and the lower part of the shank with the other hand. Co-ordinating the two hands, rotate the hip joint medially. Repeat 20-30 times. (See Fig. 17)

d. Lateral rotation of the hip joint at the head and neck of the femur. The patient

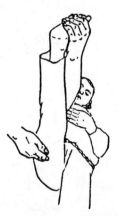

**Fig. 16   Stretch and elevate the leg and massage along the posterior aspect of the thigh with three fingers**

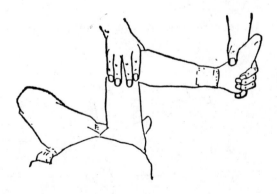

**Fig. 17   Medial rotation of hip joint**

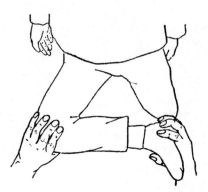

**Fig. 18    Lateral rotation of hip joint**

lies in a supine position and flexes both the hip and knee joints to 90°. The doctor holds the anterior portion of the knee joint with one hand, and the lower part of the shank with the other hand. Co-ordinating the two hands, rotate the hip joint laterally. Repeat 20-30 times. (See Fig. 18)

e. Manipulation of rectus femoris and rectus abdominis. The patient lies in a prone position. The doctor flexes the knee joint of the sick leg to 90° with the whole leg resting flat on the bed and the shank pointing inward and puts the other leg over it to form an Arabic 4. The doctor presses with one hand the gluteal region of the bad leg and massages along the rectus femoris with the other hand to relax the contracture of the rectus femoris and rectus abdominis. Repeat 20-30 times. (See Fig. 19)

f. Manipulation of tractus iliotibialis. The patient lies in a lateral recumbent posture; the doctor holds the crista iliaca with one hand and rubs down the contracted tractus iliotibialis with the fingers of the other hand until the knee touches the table. The knee joint and the hip joint of the affected leg are flexed at 90°, and the other leg is kept straight. This method applies to children aged ten and under. Repeat 20-30 times. (See Fig. 20)

Another method requires the patient to lie in the same posture but leaning

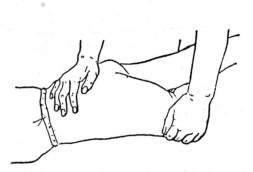

**Fig. 19    4-Form manipulation
in prone position**

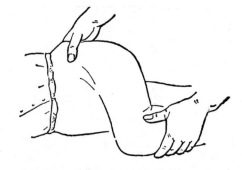

**Fig. 20    Manipulation of tractus iliotibialis**

backwards. The doctor keeps the patient in this position by leaning his chest forward against the patient's knee. He then holds the patient's knee joint with his left hand and rubs and percusses along the tractus iliotibialis 20-30 times with the fingers of the right hand to relieve contracture.

5. Orthopaedic manipulation of the ankle joint

a. Correction of foot ptosis by pressing the knee. With the knee joint in flexion to 90°, the patient lies in a supine position on the examination table. The doctor presses the upper part of the knee with one hand and uses the other hand to push the anterior portion of the ankle joint backward with the arch between the thumb and the index finger. Repeat 20-30 times. (See Fig. 21)

b. Correction of foot ptosis by pressing the foot and massaging the posterior aspect of the shank. The patient lies in a prone position, the knee joint of the affected leg flexed to 90°. The other leg remains straight. The doctor holds the front part of the foot and presses downward and adducts the index, middle and ring fingers of the other hand to massage along the gastrocnemius down to the heel tendon on the posterior aspect of the shank to correct foot ptosis. Repeat 20-30 times. (See Fig. 22)

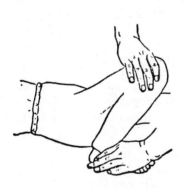

**Fig. 21    Correction of foot ptosis by pressing the knee**

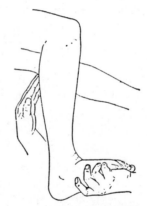

**Fig. 22    Correction of foot ptosis by pressing down on sole and massaging along the posterior aspect of the shank**

6. Orthopaedic manipulation of the foot

a. Correction of clubfoot. The patient lies in a supine position, relaxing the affected leg. The doctor holds the posterior aspect of the ankle joint with his left hand, holding the front part of the foot with his right hand and pushing it outwards to correct varus clubfoot. To correct valgus clubfoot, pull the front part of the foot inwards. Repeat 20-30 times. (See Fig. 23)

b. Correction of clawfoot. The patient lies in a supine position, flexes the knee joint of the leg with the clawfoot and puts the sole of the foot on the table. The doctor puts both hands over the tarsal sinus and presses downward suddenly, once only for each treatment. Sounds are sometimes heard in the process. Repeat the treatment until the deformity is corrected. (See Fig. 24)

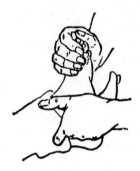

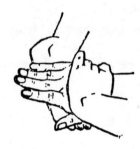

Fig. 23   Correction of clubfoot        Fig. 24   Correction of clewfoot

### 2. Orthotherapy through external fixation

When orthopaedic manipulations have reached their limit, external fixation becomes a necessity for the correction of deformed extremeties.

For drop-foot, talipes equinovarus, talipes equinovalgus and flexile contracture of the knee joint, long plaster cast with thick matting particularly over the knee joint, the anterior part of the ankle joint, the heel and the medial and lateral malleoli, is required for a period of about three weeks. If the patient complains of local pain, the cast over the painful area should be opened for examination. Short plaster cast may be used for foot deformities.

For drop-wrist, finger contracture and trouble with the supination of the forearm, long or short plaster arm cast with thick matting is required for about three weeks. The patient should extend the wrist and fingers and rotate the forearm laterally.

Frog plaster splint (abduction splint) is applied to children with congenital dislocation of the hip joint or cerebral palsy resulting in crossed legs to relax the contracture of the adductor longus and adductor magnus of the femur.

Plastic, steel-wire or wood splints can also be used for external fixation, but plaster cast is the best of all. In some cases, the patient may exercise the afflicted limb during the day and have it fixed in a plaster-of-paris bed at night.

### 3. Orthotherapy by surgery

In some cases, surgery is needed in addition to using acupressure and external fixation.

1. Lengthening of the heel tendon. When three months of continuous treatment with acupressure therapy or orthotherapy proves ineffective, surgical operation may be necessary. The lengthening of the heel tendon is best applied to patients above ten years of age, or at least above seven. It is not recommended for children under seven, because postoperative recurrence in a small child will be disastrous.

2. Scission and relaxation of the tendons of adductor longus and adductor magnus of the femur. Surgery is aimed at correcting interference with abduction of the hip joint and knock-knee caused by contracture of the adductor muscles. This is recommended when orthopaedic manipulations have proved ineffective after three months of continuous application. The patient should be at least above three or four years of

age. A second operation is in order if the first one proves unsuccessful.

3. Scission and relaxation of contracture of the tractus iliotibialis. This is best administered to children between four and five years of age when orthopaedic manipulations lasting three months or longer have failed to correct the contracture of the tractus iliotibialis, and the patient continues to walk with a limp.

## Section X

## Common Postures of the Patient During Treatment

The appropriate posture of a patient will greatly facilitate the correct location of the acupoints and acupressure manipulations. Generally speaking, a correct posture should allow the practitioner to work without hindrance and enable the patient to feel relaxed and comfortable. The postures commonly used in the clinic are as follows:

1. Sitting back in a chair: suitable for manipulating points on the face, head, neck and upper extremities. (See Fig. 25)

2. Sitting in flexion: suitable for manipulating points on the back of the head and neck, the back and upper extremities. (See Fig. 26)

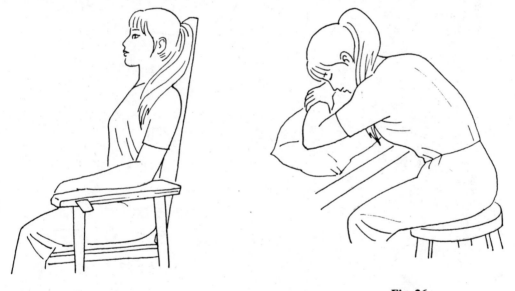

Fig. 25                    Fig. 26

3. Lateral recumbent: suitable for manipulating the points at the lateral side of the body. (See Fig. 27)

4. Supine posture: suitable for manipulating the points on the head and face, chest and abdominal regions, and areas of the anterior regions of the limbs. (See Fig. 28)

5. Prone posture: suitable for manipulating the points on the top of the head, back, lumbus, buttocks and the posterior regions of the lower limbs. (See Fig. 29)

Postures for manipulating peculiarly located acupoints are described in sections dealing with these points later in the book.

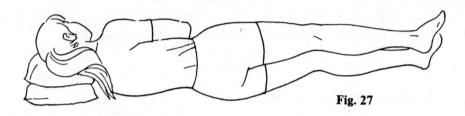

**Fig. 27**

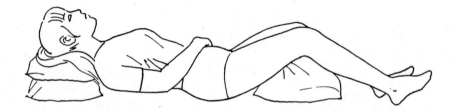

**Fig. 28**

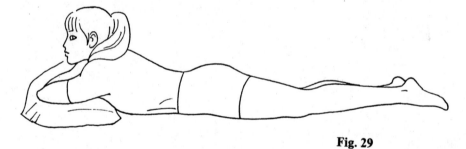

**Fig. 29**

## Section XI
## Acupoints and Stimulation-Lines

### A. Three Ways to Locate the Acupressure Points

1. Proportional measurement. The human body is divided into a number of equal measuring units, each of which is reckoned as one *cun* in length. This standard of meaurement is applicable to both adults and children of different statures. (See Fig. 30)

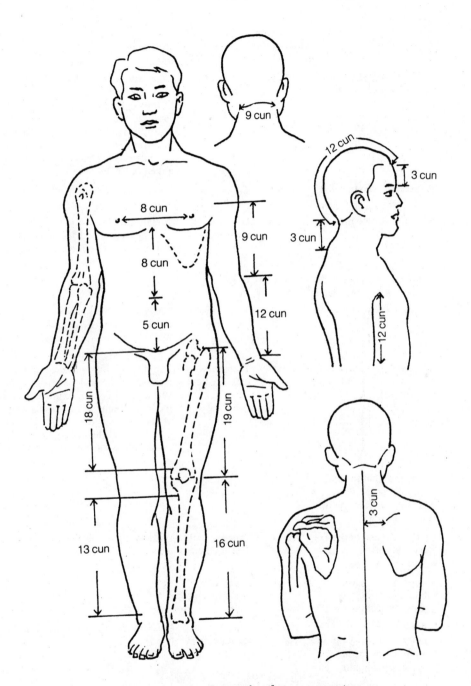

**Fig. 30 Proportional measurement**

## Standards of Proportional Measurement

| Body-part | Distance | Proportional Measurement | Method | Remarks |
|---|---|---|---|---|
| Head | From the anterior hairline to the posterior hairline | 12 *cun* | Longitudinal measurement | The distance from the glabella to the anterior hairline is taken as 3 *cun*. The distance from Dazhui (GB 14) to the posterior hairline is taken as 3 *cun*. If the anterior and posterior hairlines are indistinguishable, the distance from the glabella to Dazhui (GB 14) is then taken as 18 *cun*. |
| | Between the two mastoid bones | 9 *cun* | Transverse measurement | Transverse measurement is also used to locate other points on the head. |
| Chest and abdomen | From the sternocostal angle to the centre of the umbilicus | 8 *cun* | Longitudinal measurement | Longitudinal measurement of the chest and the hypochondriac region is generally based on the intercostal space. |
| | Between the centre of the umbilicus and the upper border of symphysis pubis | 5 *cun* | | |
| | Between the two nipples | 8 *cun* | Transverse measurement | The distance between the bilateral Quepen (ST 12) can be used as the substitute of the transverse measurement of the two nipples. |
| Back | Between the medial border of the scapula and the posterior midline | 3 *cun* | Transverse measurement | Longitudinal measurement of the back is based on the spinous processes of the vertebral column. In clinical practice, the lower angle of the scapula is at about the same level as the 7th thoracic vertebra, and the iliac spine is at about the same level as the 4th lumbar vertebra. |
| Lateral side of the chest | From the end of the axillary fold on the lateral side of the chest to the tip of the 11th rib | 12 *cun* | Longitudinal measurement | |
| Upper extremities | Between the end of the axillary fold and the transverse cubital crease | 9 *cun* | Longitudinal measurement | Used for the three Yin and three Yang meridians of the hand |
| | Between the transverse cubital crease and the transverse wrist crease | 12 *cun* | Longitudinal measurement | |
| | From the level of the upper border of the symphysis pubis to the medial epicondyle of the femur | 18 *cun* | Longitudinal measurement | Used for the three Yin meridians of the hand |
| | From the lower border of the medial condyle of the tibia to the tip of the medial malleolus | 13 *cun* | | |
| | From the prominence of | | | |

| | | | |
|---|---|---|---|
| the great trochanter to the middle of the patella | 19 *cun* | Longitudinal measurement | (1) Used for the three Yang meridians of the foot. (2) The distance from the gluteal crease to the centre of patella is taken as 14 *cun*. (3) The anterior level of the centre of the patella is at about the same level as Dubi (ST 35), and the posterior level is at about the same level as Weizhong (BL 40). |
| Between the centre of the patella and the tip of the lateral malleolus | 16 *cun* | | |
| From the tip of the lateral malleolus to the heel | 3 *cun* | | |

Some points are relatively easy to locate. For example, Danzhong (RN 17) is at the midpoint between the two nipples, and Yintang (EX-HN3) is midway between the eyebrows.

2. Finger measurement.

The length and width of the patient's fingers are taken as a standard for point location. The following three methods are commonly used.

a. Middle finger measurement. When the middle finger is flexed, the distance between the two ends of the creases of the interphalangeal joints is taken as one *cun*. This method is employed for measuring the vertical distance to locate the limb points of the Yang meridians, or for measuring the horizontal distance to locate the points on the back. (See Fig. 31)

b. Thumb measurement. The width of the interphalangeal joint of the patient's thumb is taken as one *cun*. The method is also employed for measuring the vertical distance to locate the points on the limbs. (See Fig. 31)

c. Four-finger mesurement. When the four fingers (index, middle, ring and little fingers) keep close, their width on the level of the proximal interphalangeal crease of

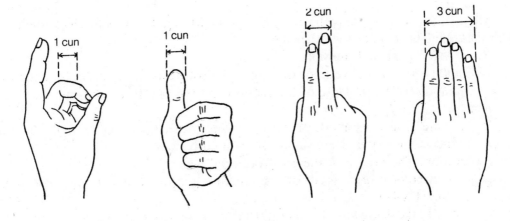

**Fig. 31   Finger measurement**

the middle finger is taken as 3 *cun*. It is used to locate the points on the limbs and in the abdominal region. (See Fig. 31)

The finger measurement is simple to apply but is not as accurate as the proportional measurement.

3. By anatomical landmarks.

The various anatomical landmarks on the body's surface are used as the basis for locating acupressure points. These landmarks fall into two categories:

a. Fixed landmark. These landmarks do not change their positions with body movement. They include the five sense organs, hair, nails, nipples, umbilicus, and prominences and depressions of the bones. They are used as points of orientation for locating acupoints. The proportional measurement is based on these anatomical landmarks. However, points that are adjacent to or right on the landmarks can be located directly. Examples are Yintang (EX-HN3) between the eyebrows, Suliao (DU 25) on the tip of the nose, and Shenque (RN 8) in the centre of the umbilicus.

b. Hidden landmarks. These landmarks will appear only when a body part is held in a specific position. For instance, when the arm is flexed and the cubital crease appears, Quchi (LI 11) can be located; and when clenching the fist and the transverse palmar crease appears, Houxi (SI 3) can be located.

## B. List of Acupoints Commonly Used in Acupressure Therapy

The following are 100 points—29 on the head; 12 on the chest and abdomen; 12 on the shoulder, neck and lumbar region; 21 on the upper extremities; 26 on the lower extremities. The code numbers of the acupoints are based on the 1990 edition of *The Location of Acupoints—State Standard of the People's Republic of China* published by the Foreign Languages Press, Beijing. Some unnumbered points are Wugong, or Martial Art points.

### 1. Points on the head and neck

1. Baihui (DU 20)

Location: On the midline of the head, 7 *cun* directly above the posterior hairline, approximately on the midpoint of the line connecting the apexes of the two auricles. (See Fig. 32)

Method: The doctor holds the patient's head with one hand and presses the point with the thumb cushion of the other hand.

Reactions: Soreness, distension.

Indications: Headache, vertigo, tinnitus, nasal obstruction, aphasia by apoplexy, coma, mental disorders, prolapse of the rectum and the uterus, cerebral palsy.

*Regional anatomy*

Vasculature: The anastomotic network formed by the superficial temporal arteries and veins and the occipital arteries and veins on both sides.

Innervation: The branch of the great occipital nerve.

Note: This point is often used for acupuncture anesthesia in cerebral operations.

2. Taiyang (EX-HN5)

Location: In the depression 1 *cun* posterior to the midpoint between the lateral end of the eyebrow and the outer corner of the eyes. (See Fig. 33)

Method: The patient sits back or lies supine. Press the point with the finger tip.

Reactions: Local soreness and distension.

Indications: Migraine, trifacial neuralgia, eye diseases, deviation of the eyes and mouth.

3. Shuaigu (GB 8)

Location: Superior to the apex of the auricle, 1.5 *cun*, within the hairline. (See Fig. 33)

Method: The doctor holds the patient's head with one hand, and presses the point with the finger cushion of the other hand's thumb or middle finger.

Reactions: Local soreness, pain, distension and dizziness.

Indications: Migraine, vertigo, vomiting, infantile convulsion, cerebral palsy.

*Regional anatomy*

Vasculature: The parietal branches of the superficial temporal artery and vein.

Innervation: The anastomotic branch of the auriculotemporal nerve and great occipital nerve.

4. Wangu (GB 12)

Location: In the depression posterior and inferior to the mastoid process. (See Fig. 33)

Method: The patient sits back in the chair or lies in prone posture. Press the point and push toward the mastoid process.

Reactions: Soreness, distension and heaviness in the head.

Indications: Headache, insomnia, swelling of the cheek, retroauricular pain, deviation of the eye and mouth, toothache, vomiting.

*Regional anatomy*

Vasculature: The posterior auricular artery and vein.

Innervation: The lesser occipital nerve.

5. Chuigen

Location: Just below lobulus auriculal. (See Fig. 33)

Method: The patient sits back or lies in the lateral recumbent position. Press the point with the tip of the thumb or index finger in the direction of the mandible.

Reactions: Local soreness, numbness diffused to the cheek, upper and lower jaw and distension in the ear.

Indications: Toothache, paralysis of facial nerve, headache.

*Regional anatomy*

The parotid situated near the point.

Innervation: The great occipital nerve.

6. Tinghui (GB 2)

Location: Anterior to the intertragic notch, at the posterior border of the condyloid process of the mandible. The point is located with the mouth open. (See Fig. 33)

Method: The doctor holds the patient's head with one hand and presses the point with the index finger of the other hand.

Reactions: Local soreness and distension diffused to the ear and face area.

Indications: Deafness, tinnitus, toothache, motor impairment of the temporomandibular joint, mumps, deviation of the eye and mouth.

*Regional anatomy*

Vasculature: The superficial temporal artery.

Innervation: The great auricular nerve and facial nerve.

7. Tinggong (SI 19)

Location: Anterior to the tragus and posterior to the condyloid process of the mandible, in the depression formed when the mouth is open. (Fig. 33)

Method: The patient sits back or lies in the lateral recumbent position. Use the tip of the thumb or index finger to lightly percuss or press the point in the direction of the mandible.

Reactions: Local soreness and distension diffused to the ear.

Indications: Deafness, tinnitus, otorrhea, motor impairment of the mandibular joint, toothache, sequela of encephalitis.

*Regional anatomy*

Vasculature: The auricular branches of the superficial temporal artery and vein.

Innervation: The branch of the facial nerve, the auriculotemporal nerve.

8. Yifeng (SJ 17)

Location: Posterior to the lobule of the ear, in the depression between the mandible and mastoid process. (Fig 33)

Method: The patient sits back or lies in the lateral recumbent position. The doctor holds the patient's head with one hand, and presses the point with the tip of the thumb of the other hand.

Reactions: Distension in the ear, warmth and distension on the head when pressure is strong.

Indications: Tinnitus, deafness, otorrhea, facial paralysis, toothache, swelling of the cheek, scrofula, trismus.

*Regional anatomy*

Vasculature: The posterior auricular artery and vein, the external jugular vein.

Innervation: The great auricular nerve; deeper, the site where the facial nerve perforates out of the stylomastoid foramen.

9. Dicang (ST 4)

Location: Lateral to the corner of the mouth, directly below Sibai (ST 2). (See Fig. 33)

Method: Press the point with the fingertip while the patient closes the mouth and clenches the teeth.

Reactions: Local soreness and distension.

Indications: Deviation of the mouth, salivation, twitching of the eyelids, facial paralysis, spasm of the facial muscles.

*Regional anatomy*

Vasculature: The facial artery and vein.

Innervation: Superficially, the branches of the facial and infraorbital nerves; deeper, the terminal branch of the buccal nerve.

10. Yintang (EX-HN3)

Location: Midway between the medial ends of the two eyebrows. (See Fig. 34)

Method: The patient sits back or lies supine. Press the point.

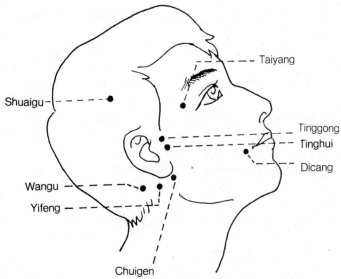

**Fig. 33**

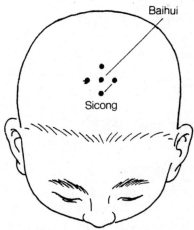

**Fig. 32**

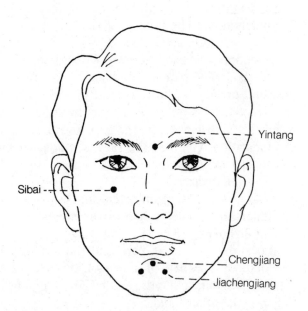

**Fig. 34**

Reactions: Local soreness, pain, numbness and distension diffused to adjacent areas.

Indications: Headache, head heaviness, epistaxis, rhinorrhea.

11. Sibai (ST 2)

Location: Below Chengqi (ST 1) in the depression at the infraorbital foramen. (See Fig. 34)

Method: Press the point with the finger pad of the thumb in the direction of the nasal bone.

Reactions: Local soreness and distension, lacrimation.

Indications: Redness, pain and itching of the eye, facial paralysis, twitching of the eyelids, pain in the face.

*Regional anatomy*

Vasculature: The branches of facial artery and vein, the infraorbital artery and vein.

Innervation: The branches of the facial nerve. The point is right on the course of the infraorbital nerve.

12. Chengjiang (RN 24)

Location: In the depression in the centre of the mentolabial groove. (See Fig. 34)

Method: Press the point with the fingertip, either downward toward the menturn tubercle or upward.

Reactions: Numbness in the lower lip and lower alveolus.

Indications: Facial puffiness, swelling of the gums, toothache, salivation, nausea, vomiting, brain trauma and sequelae of encephalitis.

*Regional anatomy*

Vasculature: The branches of the inferior labial artery and vein.

Innervation: The branch of the facial nerve.

13. Jiachengjiang (Extra 5)

Location: one *cun* lateral to Chengjiang (RN 24). (See Fig. 34)

Method: The patient sits back or lies in supine position. Press or lightly percuss the point upward with the fingertip.

Reactions: Numbness in the mouth, distension in the mandibula, salivation, soreness and distension in the ears and the superior pelpebral region.

Indications: Pain in the face, sequalae of encephalitis, deviation of the eyes and mouth, spasm of the facial muscle, alveolalgia inferior, salivation.

*Regional anatomy*

Vasculature: Mentum artery and vein.

Innervation: The branch of the mentum nerve.

14. Sizhukong (SJ 23)

Location: In the depression at the lateral end of the eyebrow. (See Fig. 35)

Method: The patient sits back or lies in supine position. The doctor holds the patient's occiput, and presses or lightly percuss the point with the tip of the index finger of the other hand.

Reactions: Local soreness and distension in the eye.

Indications: Headache, redness and pain of the eye, blurring of vision, twitching of the eyelid, toothache, facial paralysis.

*Regional anatomy*

Vasculature: The frontal branches of the superficial temporal artery and vein.

Innervation: The zygomatic branch of the facial nerve and the branch of the auriculotemporal nerve.

Muscle: Orbicular muscle of the eye under the skin.

15. Jingming (BL 1)

Location: 0.1 *cun* superior to the inner canthus. (See Fig. 35)

Method: The patient sits back or lies supine, closes his eyes and gently rolls the eyeball to the lateral side. The doctor holds the patient's head with one hand and uses the radial side of the pad of the thumb to press the point in the direction of the bridge of the nose.

Reactions: Local distension, lacrimation.

Indications: Redness, swelling and pain of the eye, itching of the canthus, lacrimation, night blindness, colour blindness, blurring of vision, myopia, strabismus, ptosis, facial paralysis, common cold, insomnia.

*Regional anatomy*

Vasculature: The angular artery and vein; deeper, in a superior position, the ophthalmic artery and vein.

Innervation: Superficially, the supratrochlear and infratrochlear nerves; deeper, the branches of the oculomotor nerve, the ophthalmic nerve.

16. Zanzhu (BL 2)

Location: On the medial extremity of the eyebrow, or on the supraorbital notch. (See Fig. 35)

Method: The patient sits back or lies supine. The doctor holds the patient's head with one hand and uses the tip of the middle finger of the other hand to press the point.

Reactions: Local soreness, numbness and distension, lacrimation.

Indications: Blurring and failing of vision, pain in the supraorbital region, lacrimation, redness, swelling and pain of the eye, twitching of the eyelids, glaucoma.

*Regional anatomy*

Vasculature: The frontal artery and vein.

Innervation: The medial branch of the frontal nerve.

17. Yuyao (EX-HN4)

Location: At the midpoint of the eyebrows. (See Fig. 35)

Method: The patient sits back or lies supine. Use the tip of the middle finger to press the point.

Reactions: Local soreness, numbness, distension, irradiation into the orbit, lacrimation.

Indications: Pain in the supraorbital region, twitching of the eyelids, cloudiness of the cornea, redness, swelling and pain of the eyes.

18. Chengqi (ST 1)

Location: With the eyes looking straight ahead, the point is directly below the pupil, between the eyeball and the infraorbital ridge. (See Fig. 35)

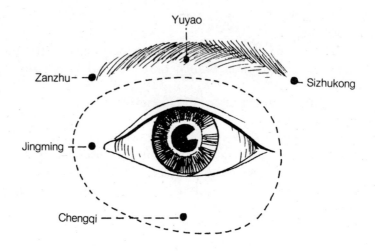

**Fig. 35**

Method: The patient sits back or lies in supine position with eyes closed. The doctor holds the patient's head with one hand, and presses the point with the tip of the thumb of the other hand. The patient tightly shuts his eyes at the same time.

Reactions: Distension in the eye, exophthalmos and lacrimation.

Indications: Redness, swelling and pain of the eye, lacrimation, night blindness, twitching of eyelids, facial paralysis.

*Regional anatomy*

Vasculature: The branches of the infraorbital and ophthalmic arteries and veins.

Innervation: The branch of the infraorbital nerve, the inferior branch of the oculomotor nerve and the muscular branch of the facial nerve.

Muscle: Orbicular muscle of the eye.

19. Yingxiang (LI 20)

Location: In the nasolabial groove, at the level of the midpoint of the lateral border of ala nasi. (See Fig. 36)

Method: Press or lightly percuss the point with the finger pad of the thumb or the index finger in the direction of the nasal bone.

Reactions: Soreness and distension.

Indications: Nasal obstruction, hyposmia, epistaxis, rhinorrhea, deviation of the mouth, itching and swelling of the face, common cold.

*Regional anatomy*

Vasculature: The facial artery and vein, the branches of the infraorbital artery and vein.

Innervation: The anastomotic branch of the facial and infraorbital nerves.

20. Suliao (DU 25)

Location: On the tip of the nose. (See Fig. 36)

Method: Press the point with the pad of the thumb in an upward direction.

Reactions: Soreness and distension in the nose, lacrimation.

Indications: Loss of consciousness, nasal obstruction, epistaxis, rhinorrhea, rosacea, sunstroke, sequelae of encephalitis.

*Regional anatomy*

Vasculature: The lateral nasal branches of the facial artery and vein.

Innervation: The external nasal branch of the anterior ethmoid nerve.

21. Bige

Location: There are three points: one directly under the nose and one on either side. (Fig. 36)

Method: The patient sits back or lies supine. Press the points with the ulnar side of the tip of the thumb.

Reactions: Numbness in the upper alveolus, distension in the head, and lacrimation.

Indications: Toothache, shock, sunstroke, sequelac of encephalitis.

*Regional anatomy*

Vasculature: Superior labial artery and vein.

Innervation: Branches of buccal nerve of facial nerve, branches of the infraorbital nerve.

22. Shanglianquan (Extra 12)

Location: one *cun* below the midpoint of the lower jaw, in the depression between the hyoid bone and the lower border of the jaw. (see Fig. 37)

Method: The patient throws back the head. The doctor's thumb or middle fingertip presses the point toward the root of the tongue.

Reactions: Numbness in the root of the tongue, salivation, inability to stick out the tongue.

Indications: Alalia, salivation with stiff tongue, difficulty in swallowing, loss of voice.

*Regional anatomy*

Vasculature: The branch to the submental area of the facial artery and vein.

Innervation: The branch of the cutaneous cervical nerve.

23. Lianquan (RN 23)

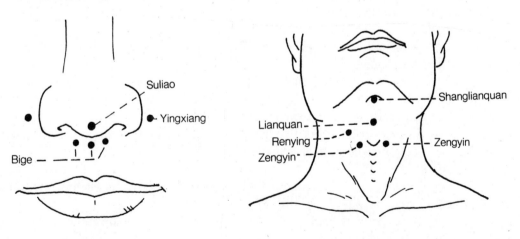

**Fig. 36**                              **Fig. 37**

Location: Above the Adam's apple, in the depression of the upper border of the hyoid bone. (See Fig. 37)

Method: The patient sits back or lies supine. Use the top of the finger. Press the point with the cushion of the finger backward and downward toward the upper border of cartilago thyroidea.

Reactions: Soreness and distension in the mandibular base, tongue root and anterior portion of the thyroid cartilage, salivation.

Indications: Swelling and pain of the subglossal region, salivation with glossoplegia, aphasia with stiffness of tongue by apoplexy, sudden hoarseness of the voice, difficulty in swallowing.

*Regional anatomy*

Vasculature: The anterior jugular vein.

Innervation: The branch of the cutaneous cervical nerve, the hypoglossal nerve, and the branch of the glossopharyngeal nerve.

24. Renying (ST 9)

Location: Level with the tip of the Adam's apple, just on the course of the common carotid artery, on the anterior border of m. sternocleidomastoideus. (See Fig. 37)

Method: The patient sits back or lies on the back.
Avoid pressing the common carotid artery which is close to the point. Use the tip or cushion of the finger to press the point.

Reactions: Depressive sensation in the throat, distension in the head and eye, numbness in the shoulder joint.

Indications: Sore throat, headache, asthma, goiter, dizziness, hypertension, sequelae of encephalitis, brain trauma, flushing of the face, cerebral dropsy.

*Regional anatomy*

Vasculature: The superior thyroid artery on the bifurcation of the internal and the external carotid artery.

Innervation: Superficially, the cutaneous cervical nerve, the cervical branch of the facial nerve; deeper, the sympathetic trunk; laterally, the descending branch of the hypoglossal nerve and the vagus nerve.

25. Zengyin (Extra 11)

Location: At the anterior aspect of the neck in the depression on either side of the thyroid cartilage. (See Fig. 37)

Method: The patient sits back or lies supine. Straighten up the patient's neck, press one point with the thumb and the other point with the index finger, then rub in a circular movement without lifting the fingers.

Reactions: Local soreness and distension and feeling of obstruction in the larynx.

Indications: Dysphasia, partial loss of voice.

26. Tianzhu (BL 10)

Location: 1.3 *cun* lateral to Yamen (DU 15), within the posterior hairline, on the lateral aspect of m. trapezius. (See Fig. 38)

Method: The patient sits back or lies prone. Use the pad of the finger to press the point in the direction of the orbit on the opposite side.

Reactions: Soreness and numbness in the neck, distension in the head.

Indications: Headache, nasal obstruction, sore throat, neck rigidity, pain in the shoulder and back, paralysis caused by celebrosis, neurasthenia, eye diseases.

*Regional anatomy*

Vasculature: The occipital artery and vein.

Innervation: The great occipital nerve.

27. Fengchi (GB 20)

Location: In the depression between the upper portion of m. sternocleidomastoideus and m. trapezius. (See Fig. 38)

Method: The patient sits back or lies in the lateral recumbent position. Use the pad of the middle finger to press or percuss the point in the direction of the orbit on the opposite side.

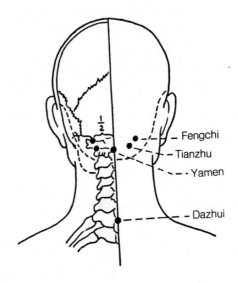

Fig. 38

Reactions: Soreness and distension in the posterior portion of the neck and in some cases, distension and sensation of protopsis in the eye.

Indications: Headache, vertigo, insomnia, neurasthenia, sequelae of encephalitis and brain trauma, cerebral agenesis.

*Regional anatomy*

Vasculature: The branches of the occipital artery and vein.

Innervation: The branch of the lesser occipital nerve.

28. Yamen (DU 15)

Location: 0.5 *cun* directly above the midpoint of the posterior hairline, in the depression below the spinous process of the first cervical vertebra. (See Fig. 38)

Method: The patient sits back. Use the finger tip to press the point, and rub lightly in a circular movement.

Reactions: Local soreness, numbness, distension.

Indications: Mental disorders, deafness and mute syndrome, sudden hoarseness of voice, stiffness of the tongue and aphasia, occipital headache, neck rigidity.

*Regional anatomy*

Vasculature: The branches of the occipital artery and vein.

Innervation: The third occipital nerve.

Other reference: Needling the Yamen point will increase the total amount of white blood cells and neutrophils and decrease the number of the lymphocytes, and may improve the hematopoietic function of bone marrow.

29. Dazhui (DU 14)

Location: Below the spinous processes of the seventh cervical vertebra, approximately at the level of the shoulders. (See Fig. 38)

Method: Press the point with the fingertip and knead in a circular movement.

Reactions: Local soreness, numbness, distension.

Indications: Neck pain and rigidity, sunstroke, fabrile diseases, epilepsy, afternoon fever, asthma, back stiffness.

*Regional anatomy*

Vasculature: The branch of the transverse cervical artery.

Innervation: The posterior ramus of the eighth cervical nerve and the medial branch of the posterior ramus of the first thoracic nerve.

## 2. Points on the thoracic and abdominal regions

1. Tiantu (RN 22)

Location: In the centre of the suprasternal fossa. (See Fig. 39)

Method: The patient sits erect or lies supine. Press the point with the pad of the finger.

Reactions: Local soreness, distension, stuffiness in the chest.

Indications: Asthma, cough, sore throat, dry throat, hiccup, sudden hoarseness of the voice, difficulty in swallowing, sequelae of encephalitis, anomic aphasia.

*Regional anatomy*

Vasculature: Superficially, the jugular arch and the branch of the inferior thyroid artery; deeper, the trachea; in an inferior position, at the posterior aspect of the sternum, the innominate vein and aortic arch.

Innervation: The anterior branch of the supraclavicular nerve.

Muscle: In the midpoint of the sternocleidomastoid muscle; deeper, sternohyoid and sternothyroideus muscles.

2. Quepen (ST 12)

Location: In the midpoint of the supraclavicular fossa, 4 *cun* lateral to the Ren Meridian. (See Fig. 39)

Method: The patient sits erect or lies supine. Percuss or press the point and knead back and forth.

Reactions: Local soreness, pain, distension and numbness diffused to the shoulder or fingers.

Indications: Paralysis of upper extremities, numbness of arms, hypertension, headache, toothache.

*Regional anatomy*

Vasculature: In a superior position, the transverse cervical artery.

Innervation: Superficially, the intermediate supraclavicular nerve; deeper, the supraclavicular portion of brachial plexus.

3. Jiuwei (RN 15)

Location: Below the xyphoid process, 7 *cun* above the umbilicus; locate the point in supine position with the arms uplifted. (Fig. 39)

Method: The patient lies in supine position and breathes diaphragmatically. Percuss or press the point in a downward direction in time with the heaving abdomen.

Reactions: Warmth and distension in the abdomen.

Indications: Pain in the cardiac region and the stomach, nausea, digestive disorders, epilepsy.

*Regional anatomy*

Vasculature: The superior epigastric artery and vein.

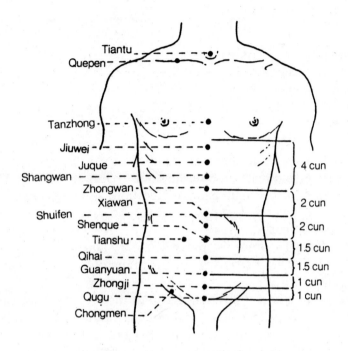

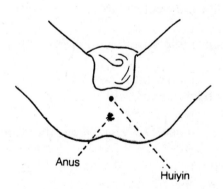

**Fig. 39**

Innervation: The anterior cutaneous branch of the seventh intercostal nerve.

4. Juque (RN 14)

Location: On the midline of the abdomen. 6 *cun* above the umbilicus. (See Fig. 39)

Method: Same as Jiuwei (RN 15).

Indications: Same as Jiuwei (RN 15).

*Regional anatomy*: Same as Jiuwei (RN 15).

Note: The left lobe of the liver is located deep under this point. Do not press too hard.

5. Shenque (RN 8)

Location: In the centre of the umbilicus. (See Fig. 39)

The method and reactions are the same as Jiuwei (RN 15). Do not press too hard.

Indications: Abdominal pain, indigestion, borborygmus, abdominal distension, unchecked diarrhoea.

*Regional anatomy*

Vasculature: The inferior epigastric artery and vein.

Innervation: The anterior cutaneous branch of the tenth intercostal nerve.

6. Tianshu (ST 25)

Location: In a lateral position, 2 *cun* to the centre of the umbilicus. (See Fig. 39)

Method: The patient lies in supine position and breathes diaphragmatically. During inhalation, press the point in a downward direction.

Reactions: Warmth, distension and numbness in the abdomen; in some cases, the sensation is diffused to the perineal region.

Indications: Abdominal pain and distension, borborygmus, pain around the umbilicus, indigestion, incontinence, diarrhoea, dysentery, irregular menstruation.

*Regional anatomy*

Vasculature: The branches of the tenth intercostal and inferior epigastric arteries and veins.

Innervation: The branch of the tenth intercostal nerve.

Muscle: The corresponding rectus abdominis muscle.

7. Qihai (RN 6)

Location: On the midline of the abdomen, 1.5 *cun* below the umbilicus. (See Fig. 39)

Method: The patient lies in supine position and breathes diaphragmatically. During inhalation, press the point in a downward direction.

Reactions: Warmth, distension, numbness in the abdomen, and in some patients, the sensation is diffused to the perineal region.

Indications: Abdominal pain, enuresis, nocturnal emission, impotence, diarrhoea, dysentery, uterine bleeding, irregular menstruation, dysmenorrhea, amenorrhea, mobid leukorrhea, postpartum hemorrhage.

*Regional anatomy*

Vasculature: The branches of superficial epigastric artery and vein, and the branches of inferior epigastric artery and vein.

Innervation: The branch of the iliohypogastric nerve.

8. Guanyuan (RN 4)

Location: On the midline of the abdomen, 3 *cun* below the umbilicus. (See Fig. 39)

Method: The patient lies supine. Press with the tip or pad of the finger.

Reactions: Warmth, distension, numbness in the abdomen and the sensation may be diffused to the perineal region.

Indications: Enuresis, nocturnal emission, frequency of urination, fecal and urinary incontinence, irregular menstruation, morbid leukorrhea, dysmenorrhea, uterine bleeding, postpartum hemorrhage, lower abdominal pain, abdominal distension, indigestion, diarrhea, prolapse of the rectum, impotence.

*Regional anatomy*

Vasculature: The branches of superficial epigastric artery and vein, and the branches of inferior epigastric artery and vein.

Innervation: The branch of the iliohypogastric nerve.

Note: The patient should urinate before treatment.

9. Zhongji (RN 3)

Location: On the midline of the abdomen, 4 *cun* below the umbilicus. (See Fig. 39)

Method: The patient lies supine. Press the point with the fingertip.

Reactions: Same as Guanyuan (RN 4).

Indications: Same as Guanyuan (RN 4).

10. Qugu (RN 2)

Location: On the midpoint of the upper border of the symphysis pubis. (See Fig. 39)

Method: The patient lies supine. Press or percuss the point.

Reactions: Local pain, distension, numbness.

Indications: Retention and dribbling of urine, enuresis, nocturnal emission, impotence, morbid leukorrhea, irregular menstruation, dysmenorrhea, urinary incontinence.

*Regional anatomy*

Vasculature: The branches of the inferior epigastric artery and the obturator artery.

Note: Great care should be taken when this treatment is given to pregnant women.

Innervation: The branch of the iliohypogastric nerve.

11. Chongmen (SP 12)

Location: Superior to the lateral end of the inguinal groove, on the lateral side of the femoral artery, at the level of the upper border of symphysis pubis, 3.5 *cun* lateral to Qugu (RN 2). (See Fig. 39)

Method: The patient lies in supine position. Press the point with the fingertip.

Reactions: Local pain, distension, soreness diffused to adjacent areas.

Indications: Hernia, dysuria, enuresis, spermatitis, orchiopathy.

*Regional anatomy*

Vasculature: On the medial side, the femoral artery.

Innervation: Just where the femoral nerve traverses, and the iliohypogastric nerve.

12. Huiyin (RN 1)

Location: Between the anus and the scrotum in males and between the anus and the posterior labial commissure in females. (Fig. 39)

Method: The patient lies in bed. Press the point perpendicularly with the fingertip.

Reactions: Local soreness, distension, numbness.

Indications: Vaginitis, retention of urine, hemorrhoid, nocturnal emission, enuresis, irregular menstruation, prolapse of uterus.

*Regional anatomy*

Vasculature: The branches of the perineal artery and vein.

Innervation: The branch of the perineal nerve.

### 3. Points on the shoulder, back and lumbar region

1. Jianjing (GB 21)

Location: Midway between Dazhui (DU 14) and the acromion, at the highest point of the shoulder. (See Fig.40)

Method: The patient sits back. Percuss or press the point and knead back and forth.

Reactions: Soreness, heaviness in the shoulder.

Indications: Pain and rigidity of the neck, pain in the shoulder and back, motor impairment of the arm, hypertension.

*Regional anatomy*

Vasculature: The transverse cervical artery and vein.

Innervation: The posterior branch of the subclavicular nerve, the accessory nerve.

2. Bingfeng (SI 12)

Location: In the centre of the suprascapular fossa, directly above Tianzong (SI 11). When the arm is lifted, the point is at the site of the depression. (See Fig. 40)

Method: The patient sits back. Percuss or press the point.

Reactions: Local soreness and distension.

Indications: Pain in the scapular region, numbness and aching of the upper extremities, motor impairment of the shoulder and arm.

*Regional anatomy*

Vasculature: The suprascapular artery and vein.

Innervation: The lateral suprascapular nerve and accessory nerve: deeper, the suprascapular nerve.

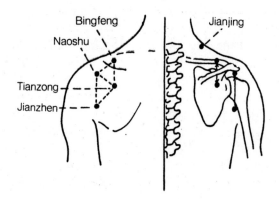

**Fig. 40**

3. Tianzong (SI 11)

Location: In the infrascapular fossa, at the junction of the upper and middle third of the distance between the lower border of the scapular spine and the inferior angle of the scapula. (See Fig. 40)

Method: The patient sits back. Percuss or press the point and knead back and forth.

Reactions: Soreness, numbness, heaviness in the upper arm.

Indications: Pain in the scapular region, pain in the lateroposterior aspect of the elbow and arm.

*Regional anatomy*

Vasculature: The muscular branches of the circumflex scapular artery and vein.

Innervation: The suprascapular nerve.

4. Naoshu (SI 10)

Location: When the arm is adducted, th point is directly above Jianzhen (SI 9), in the depression inferior and lateral to the scapular spine. (See Figs. 40 & 41)

Method: The patient sits or lies prone. Percuss and press the point.

Reactions: Local soreness, numbness, distension.

Indications: Swelling of the shoulder, aching and weakness of the shoulder and arm.

*Regional anatomy*

Vasculature: The posterior circumflex humeral artery and vein; deeper, the suprascapular artery and vein.

Innervation: The posterior cutaneous nerve of the arm, the axillary nerve; deeper, the suprascapular nerve.

5. Jianzhen (SI 9)

Location: Posterior and inferior to the shoulder jont. When the arm is adducted, the point is one *cun* above the posterior end of the axillary fold. (See Fig. 40)

Method: The patient sits and drops the arms. Percuss and press the point.

Reactions: Local soreness, distension, numbness.

Indications: Pain in the scapular region, motor impairment of the hand and arm.

*Regional anatomy*

Vasculature: The circumflex scapular artery and vein.

Innervation: The branch of the axillary nerve; deeper in the superior aspect, the radial nerve.

6. Fufen (BL 41)

Location: 3 *cun* lateral to the Du Meridian, at the level of the lower border of the spinous process of the second thoracic vertebra, on the spinal border of the scapula. (See Fig. 41)

Method: The patient sits or lies prone. Percuss and press the point, or press the point and knead back and forth.

Reactions: Distension, soreness, stuffiness in the chest, difficulty in breathing.

Indications: Stiffness and pain of the shoulder, back and neck, numbness of the elbow and arm.

*Regional anatomy*

Vasculature: The descending branch of the transverse cervical artery, the posterior branches of the intercostal artery and vein.

Innervations: The lateral branches of the posterior rami of the first and second thoracic nerves; deeper, the dorsal scapular nerve.

Muscle: The border of musculi trapezius and rhomboideus.

7. Fengmen (BL 12)

Location: 1.5 *cun* lateral to the Du Meridian, at the level of the lower border of the spinous process of the second thoracic vertebra. (See Fig. 41)

Method: The patient sits or lies prone. Lightly percuss and press the point, press the point and knead back and forth.

Reactions: Local soreness, numbness, distension. Difficulty in breathing during strong stimulation.

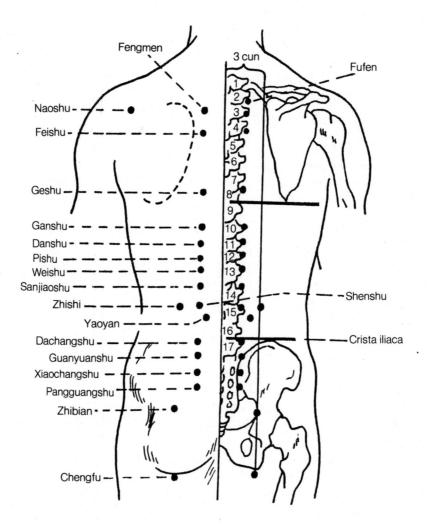

**Fig. 41**

Indications: Common cold, cough, fever and headache, neck rigidity, backache.
*Regional anatomy*
Vasculature: The medial cutaneous branches of the posterior branches of the intercostal artery and vein.
Innervation: Superficially, the medial cutaneous branches of the posterior rami of the second and third thoracic nerves; deeper, their lateral cutaneous branches.

8. Geshu (BL 17)
Location: 1.5 *cun* lateral to the Du Meridian, at the level of the lower border of the spinous process of the seventh thoracic vertebra. (See Fig. 41)
Method: The patient sits or lies prone. Percuss lightly or press the point.
Reactions: Local soreness, tenderness, sometimes conducted to the epigastric region.
Indications: Stomachache, nausea, vomiting, hiccup, belching, cough.
*Regional anatomy*
Vasculature: The medial branches of the posterior branches of the intercostal artery and vein.
Innervation: The medial branches of the posterior rami of the seventh and eighth thoracic nerves; deeper, their lateral branches.

9. Shenshu (BL 23)
Location: 1.5 *cun* lateral to the lower border of the spinous process of the second lumbar vertebra. (See Fig. 41)
Method: The patient lies in prone position. Percuss and press the point.
Reactions: Local soreness, distension conducted downward or to the abdomen.
Indications: Nocturnal emission, impotence, enuresis, irregular menstruation, leukorrhea, low back pain, weakness of the knee, blurring of vision, dizziness, tinnitus.
*Regional anatomy*
Vasculature: The posterior branches of the second lumbar artery and vein.
Innervation: The lateral branch of the posterior ramus of the first lumbar nerve; deeper, its lateral branch.

10. Yaoyan (EX-B7)
Location: In the depression lateral to the interspace between the spinous processes of the fourth and fifth lumbar vertebrae. The point is located in prone position. (See Fig. 41)
Method: The patient lies prone. Percuss and press the point or press the point and knead back and forth.
Reactions: Local soreness, distension, pain conducted to the legs.
Indications: Lumbar pain, enuresis, frequent urination, irregular menstruation, hypogastralgia, indigestion, ischidynia.
*Regional anatomy*
Vasculature: Posterior branch of the second lumbar artery and vein.
Innervation: Posterior cutaneous branch of the first lumbar nerve; deeper, the lateral branch of the posterior branch of the first lumbar nerve, and the lateral branch of the posterior branch of the thoracic nerve.
Muscle: Musculi latissimus dorsi and sacrospinalis.

11. Guanyuanshu (BL 26)

Location: 1.5 *cun* lateral to the lower border of the spinous process of the fifth lumbar vertebra. (See Fig. 41)

Method: The patient sits or lies prone. Percuss and press the point.

Reactions: Local soreness, distension, numbness conducted to the hip joint.

Indications: Low back pain, abdominal distension, diarrhoea, enuresis, sciatica, frequent urination, paralysis of lower extremity.

*Regional anatomy*

Vasculature: The posterior branches of the lowest lumbar artery and vein.

Innervation: The posterior ramus of the fifth lumbar nerve.

Muscle: Sacrospinalis muscle.

12. Pangguangshu (BL 28)

Location: 1.5 *cun* lateral to the Du Meridian, at the level of the second posterior sacral foramen. (See Fig. 41)

Method: The patient lies prone or stands. Percuss and press the point.

Reactions: Local distension, soreness sometimes conducted to the sacral and coccygeal regions.

Indications: Retention of urine, enuresis, frequent urination, constipation, stiffness and pain of the lower back.

*Regional anatomy*

Vasculature: The posterior branches of the lateral sacral artery and vein.

Innervation: The lateral branches of the posterior rami of the first and second sacral nerves.

### 4. Points on the upper extremities

1. Jianyu (LI 15)

Location: Anteroinferior to the acromion, on the upper portion of m. deltoideus. When the arm is in full abduction, the point is in the depression appearing at the anterior border of the acromioclavicular joint. (See Fig. 42)

Method: The patient sits upright. Percuss the point or press and knead the point back and forth.

Reactions: Soreness and distension around the shoulder joint.

Indications: Pain in the shoulder and arm, motor impairment of the upper extremities.

*Regional anatomy*

Vasculature: The posterior circumflex artery and vein.

Innervation: The lateral supraclavicular nerve and axillary nerve.

2. Hegu (LI 4)

Location: On the dorsum of the hand, between the first and second metacarpal bones, approximately in the middle of the second metacarpal bone on the radial side. Or, place the transverse crease of the interphalangeal joint of the thumb in a position coincident with the margin of the web between the thumb and the index finger of the other hand. The point is where the tip of the thumb touches. (See Fig. 42)

Method: Press, percuss or press and knead the point in the direction of the second ossa metacarpi.

Reactions: Local soreness, distension, numbnesss in the hand conducted upward along the radial side of the forearm.

Indications: Headache, toothache, hypertention, impairment of the upper limbs.

*Regional anatomy*

Vasculature: The venous network of the dorsum of the hand.

Innervation: The superficial ramus of the radial nerve.

Note: Stimulating the Hegu point may cause miscarriage. Do not apply it to women during pregnancy.

3. Zhangjian

Location: Between the spaces of the caputs of II-III, III-IV and IV-V ossa metacarpi on the dorsal aspect of the hand, about 0.3 *cun* above the metacarpophalangeal joints. (See Fig. 42)

Method: Percuss, press or press and knead the points.

Reactions: Local soreness, distension, numbness conducted to the fingers and forearms.

Indications: Paralysis of the upper extremities, numbness of the arm and hand, sequelae of cerebral birth injury, cerebral trauma, encephalitis and neuraxsthenia.

*Regional anatomy*

Vasculature: Metacarpal dorsal artery, dorsal venous network of the hand.

Innervation: The superficial branch of the radial nerve, dorsal branch of the ulnar nerve.

Muscles: The points located between the musculi interossi dorsalis.

4. Quchi (LI 11)

Location: When the elbow is flexed, the point is in the depression at the lateral end of the transverse cubital crease. (See Fig. 42)

Method: Press or percuss the point, or press and knead the point back and forth.

Reactions: Local soreness, distension, numbness conducted to the wrist.

Indications: hypertension, pain in the arm and shoulder, paralysis of the upper extremities, disease of the elbow and its surrounding cartilage.

*Regional anatomy*

Vasculature: The branches of the radial recurrent artery and vein.

Innervation: The posterior antebrachial cutaneous nerve; deeper, on the medial side, the radial nerve.

5. Jihui

Location: One *cun* medial to Quchi (LI 11) point. (See Fig. 42)

Method: Percuss or press the point.

Reactions: Soreness, distension and numbness in the forearm.

Indications: Headache, toothache, paralysis of the arm, sequelae of eucephalitis.

*Regional anatomy*

Vasculature: The branches of the radial recurrent artery and vein.

Innervation: The deep branch of the radial nerve, cutaneous brachial lateral nerve.

Muscles: Musculi brachioradialis and extensor carpi radialis longus.

6. Shousanli ( LI 10 )

Location: On the line joining Yangxi (LI 5) and Quchi (LI 11), 2 *cun* below Quchi

(LI 11). (See Fig. 42)

Method: Percuss or press the point, or press the point and knead back and forth.

Reactions: Local soreness, numbness, distension conducted to the middle finger.

Indications: Numbness and pain in the arm, paralysis of the upper extremities.

*Regional anatomy*

Vasculature: The branches of the radial recurrent artery and vein.

Innervation: The posterior antebrachial cutaneous nerve and the deep ramus of the radial nerve.

Muscle: Extensor carpi radialis longus.

7. Waiguan (SJ 5)

Location: 2 *cun* above Yangchi (SJ 4), between the radius and ulna. (See Fig. 42)

Method: Same as Sidu (SJ 9).

Indications: Febrile diseases, headache, deafness, tinnitus, pain in the hypochondriac region, motor impairment of the elbow and arm.

*Regional anatomy*

Vasculature: Deeper, the posterior and anterior antebrachial interosseous arteries and veins.

Innervation: The posterior antebrachial cutaneous nerve; deeper, the posterior interosseous nerve and the anterior interosseous nerve.

Acupuncture analgesia: Needling Waiguan (SJ 5) through to Neiguan (PC 6) (see Fig. 44) produces analgesia for surgeries such as cataractopiesis, pneumonectomy and operations on the esophagus, pelvis renalis and ureter.

8. Yangchi (SJ 4)

Location: On the transverse crease of the dorsum of the wrist, in the depression lateral to the tendon of m. extensor digitorum communis. (See Fig. 42)

Method: Percuss, press or press and knead the point in the ulnar direction.

Reactions: Local soreness, distension conducted to the fingers.

Indications: Headache, toothache, damage to the wrist joint and its surrounding cartilage, paralysis of the upper extremities.

*Regional anatomy*

Vasculature: The dorsal venous network of the wrist and the posterior carpal artery.

Innervation: The terminal branch of the posterior antebrachial cutaneous nerve and the dorsal branch of the ulnar nerve.

9. Sidu (SJ 9)

Location: On the lateral side of the forearm, 5 *cun* below the olecranon, between the radius and ulna. (See Fig. 42)

Method: Percuss, press or press and knead the point.

Reactions: Local soreness, distension, numbness conducted to the posterior aspect of the forearm.

Indications: Toothache, pain in the forearm, muscle atrophy of the forearm.

*Regional anatomy*

Vasculature: The posterior antebrachial interosseous artery and vein.

Innervation: The posterior and medial antebrachial cutaneous nerves; deeper, the posterior and anterior interosseous nerves.

10. Yangxi (LI 5)

Location: On the radial side of the wrist. When the thumb is tilted upward, it is in the depression between the tendons of m. extensor pollicis longus and brevis. (See Fig. 43)

Method: Press or press and knead the point.

Reactions: Local soreness, distension, numbness conducted to the thumb, index finger and the radial side of the forearm, weakness in the thumb and index finger, inability to clench a fist and hold things firmly.

Indications: Headache, deafness, pain in the wrist, spasm of the thumb.

*Regional anatomy*

Vasculature: The cephalic vein, the radial artery and its dorsal carpal branch.

Innervation' The superficial ramus of the radial nerve.

11. Binao (LI 14)

Location: 7 *cun* above Quchi (LI 11) on the radial side of the humerus, superior to the lower end of m. deltoideus. It is on the line joining Quchi (LI 11) and Jianyu (LI 15). (See Fig. 43)

Method: Percuss, press and /or press and knead the point back and forth.

Reactions: Local soreness, distension, numbness, warmth in the upper arm.

Indications: Pain in the shoulder and arm, rigidity of the neck, scrofula, paralysis of the arm.

*Regional anatomy*

Vasculature: The branches of posterior circumflex humeral artery and vein, the deep brachial artery and vein.

Innervation: The posterior brachial cutaneous nerve; deeper, the radial nerve.

Note: Needling Binao point through to Jianyu point is often done as acupuncture anesthesia for pneumonectomy and surgery of the esophagus.

12. Naohui (SJ 13)

Location: On the line joining Jianliao (SJ 14) and the olecranon, 3 *cun* below Jianliao (SJ 14) on the posterior border of m. deltoideus. (See Fig. 43)

Method and Reactions: See Binao (LI 14).

Indications: Pains in the shoulder and arm, eye diseases, paralysis of the radial nerve, numbness of the upper arm.

*Regional anatomy*

Vasculature: The median collateral artery and vein.

Innervation: The posterior brachial cutaneous nerve, the muscular branch of the radial nerve; deeper, the radial nerve.

13. Jianliao (SJ 14)

Location: Posterior and inferior to the acromion, in the depression about 1 *cun* posterior to Jianyu (LI 15) when the arm is abducted. (See Fig. 43)

Method: Percuss, press and/or press and knead the point back and forth.

Reactions: Local soreness, distension, numbness.

Indications: Pain and motor impairment of the shoulder and upper arm.

*Regional anatomy*

Vasculature: The muscular branch of the posterior circumflex humeral artery.

Innervation: The muscular branch of the axillary nerve.

14. Zhima

Location: One *cun* below the midpoint of the axillary fossa on the ulnar side of musculus biceps brachii. (See Fig. 44)

Method: Press with the fingertip and knead the point back and forth, or press the point with the thumb and the other four fingers and pinch and quickly lift the muscle between the medial border of the short head of the biceps brachii muscle and the triceps brachii muscles.

Reactions: Local soreness, numbness conducted to the fingertips.

Indications: Paralysis of the arm, numbness of the arm, common cold, headache, hypertension.

*Regional anatomy*

Vasculature: The brachial artery.

Innervation: The median nerve and ulnar nerve.

Muscle: Musculi bicep brachii and tricep brachii.

15. Xiabai (LU 4)

Location: On the medial aspect of the upper arm on the radial side of musculus biceps brachii, 4 *cun* below the end of anterior axillary stria. (See Fig. 44)

Method: Percuss, press and/or press the point back and forth.

Reactions: Local soreness and distension conducted downward.

Indications: Cough, fullness in the chest, short breath, pain in the medial aspect of the upper arm, muscular atrophy of the upper arm.

*Regional anatomy*

Vasculature: The cephalic vein and muscular branches of the brachial artery and vein.

Innervation: The lateral brachial cutaneous nerve at the place where the musculocutaneous nerve passes through.

16. Shaohai (HT 3)

Location: When the elbow is flexed into a right angle, the point is in the depression between the medial end of the transverse cubital crease and the medial epicondyle of the humerus. (See Fig. 44)

Method: Percuss or press the point, or press and knead the point back and forth.

Reactions: Soreness, numbness conducted downward to the ring and little fingers; upward to the medial side of the upper arm; paralysis of the upper extremities.

Indications: Cardiac pain, spasmodic pain and numbness of the hand and arm, tremor of the hand, scrofula, pain in the axilla, elbow and hypochondriac region.

*Regional anatomy*

Vasculature: The basilic vein, the inferior ulnar collateral artery, the ulnar recurrent artery and vein.

Innervation: The medial antebrachial cutaneous nerve, median nerve.

17. Ximen (PC 4)

Location: 5 *cun* above the transverse crease of the wrist, between the tendons of m. palmaris longus and m. flexor carpi radialis. (See Fig. 44)

Method: Percuss or press the point, or press the point and knead back and forth.

Reactions: Local soreness, distension, numbness conducted to the fingertips, sensation of heaviness when extending the wrist joint.

Indications: Dizziness, palpitation, nausea, paralysis of the upper extremeties.

*Regional anatomy*

Vasculature: The median artery and vein; deeper, the anterior interosseous artery and vein.

Innervation: The medial antebrachial cutaneous nerve; deeper, the median nerve; deepest, the anterior interosseous nerve.

18. Daling (PC 7)

Location: In the middle of the transverse crease of the wrist, between the tendons of m. palmaris longus and m. flexor carpi radialis. (See Fig. 44)

Method: Press the point with the pad or tip of the thumb. Press the dorsal aspect of the wrist with the tip of the middle finger at the same time.

Reactions: Local soreness, distension, numbness conducted to the fingers.

Indications: Numbness or paralysis of the arm, damage to the wrist joint and its surrounding cartilage.

*Regional anatomy*

Vasculature: The palmar arterial and venous network of the wrist.

Innervation: The medial cutaneous nerves; deeper, the median nerve.

19. Neiguan (PC 6)

Location: 2 *cun* above the transverse crease of the wrist, between the tendons of m. palmaris longus and m. flexor radialis. (See Fig. 44)

Method: Press or press and knead with the tip of the thumb; at the same time press the posterior aspect of the forearm with the index and middle fingers.

Reactions: Local soreness, distension, numbness conducted to the fingers.

Vasculature: See Ximen (PC 4)

Innervation: See Ximen (PC 4)

20. Zhijiagen

Location: On the nail-fold of the thumb, and the index, middle, ring and little fingers. (See Fig. 45)

Method: Hold the patient's finger with the thumb on top and the index finger underneath and pinch the points with the tip of the thumb one after another. Pinch each point 3-5 times.

Reactions: Local pain, soreness, heat.

Indications: Paralysis or numbness of the upper extremities, vomiting, common cold, shock, dizziness.

*Regional anatomy*

Vasculature: The network of the digital palmar propio-artery and vein, and the digital dorsal artery and vein.

Innervation: The digital palmar proprio-nerve and the digital dorsal nerve from the ulnar and median nerves.

21. Zhiguanjie

Location: At the transverse crease of the proximal and distal interphalangeal joints

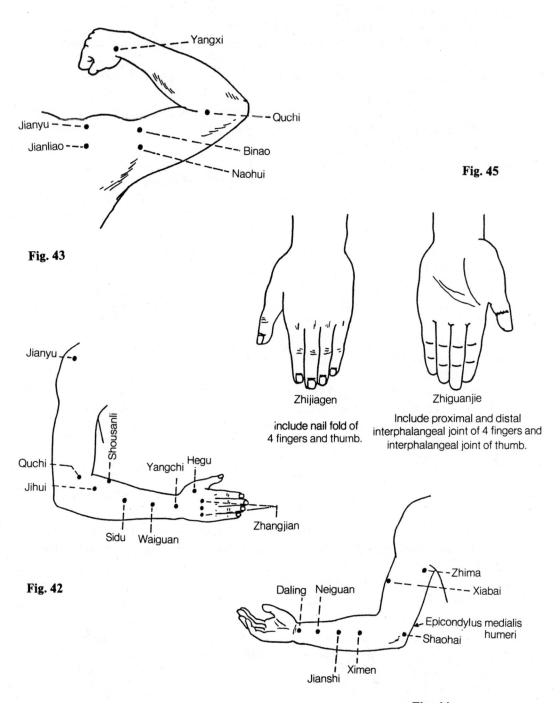

Fig. 43

Fig. 45

Fig. 42

Zhijiagen

**include nail fold of
4 fingers and thumb.**

Zhiguanjie

**Include proximal and distal
interphalangeal joint of 4 fingers and
interphalangeal joint of thumb.**

Fig. 44

of the index, middle, ring and little fingers, and the interphalangeal joint of the thumb, at the palmar aspect. (See Fig. 45)

Method: Pinch the points in the same way as for Zhijiagen, point 20.

Indications: Paralysis or numbness of the upper extremities, injuries of the ulnar, radial and median nerves, shock, vomiting, dizziness, common cold.

*Regional anatomy*: Same as 20. Zhijiagen.

The proximal interphalangeal joints are those between the proximal phalanges and the middle phalanges; the distal interphalangeal joints are those between the middle phalanges and the distal phalanges.

### 5. Points on the lower extremities

1. Huantiao (GB 30)

Location: At the junction of the middle and lateral third of the distance between the great trochanter and the hiatus of the sacrum. When locating the point, put the patient in a lateral recumbent position with the thigh flexed. (See Fig. 46)

Method: Percuss, press or press and knead the point.

Reactions: Local soreness, distension conducted to the popliteal fossa or the calcaneal region.

Indications: Pain of the lumbar region, injury of the hip joint and its adjacent cartilage, paralysis of the lower limbs, hemiplegia, ischialgia.

*Regional anatomy*

Vasculature: Medially, the inferior gluteal artery and vein.

Innervation: The inferior cluneal cutaneous nerve, the inferior gluteal nerve; deeper, the sciatic nerve.

2. Fengshi (GB 31)

Location: On the midline of the lateral aspect of the thigh, 7 *cun* above the transverse popliteal crease. When the patient is standing erect with the hands close to the sides, the point is where the tip of the middle finger touches. (See Fig. 46)

Method: Percuss, press or press and knead the point.

Reactions: Local soreness, distension, numbness conducted to the lateral aspect of the thigh.

Indications: Atrophy, numbness and paralysis of the lower limbs, hemiparalysis.

*Regional anatomy*

Vasculature: The muscular branches of the lateral circumflex femoral artery and vein.

Innervation: The lateral femoral cutaneous nerve, the muscular branch of the femoral nerve.

3. Yanglingquan (GB 34)

Location: In the depression anterior and inferior to the head of the fibula. (See Fig. 46)

Method: The patient sits erect or lies supine. Percuss or press the point.

Reactions: Local soreness, distension.

Indications: Paralysis of the lower extremities, swelling and pain of the knee.

*Regional anatomy*

Vasculature: The inferior lateral genicular artery and vein.

Innervation: Just where the common peroneal nerve bifurcates into the superficial and deep peroneal nerves.

Muscles: Musculi peroneus longus, extensor digitorum longus.

Note: Avoid injuring the peroneus communis nerve during clinical practice.

4. Yangjiao (GB 35)

Location: 7 *cun* above the tip of the external malleolus, on the posterior border of the fibula. (See Fig. 46)

Method: Percuss, press or press and knead the point.

Reactions: Local soreness, distension conducted to the lateral side of the malleola and foot.

Indications: Numbness of the leg, weak ankle, pain in the knee joint.

*Regional anatomy*

Vasculature: The branches of the peroneal artery and vein.

Innervation: The lateral sural cutaneous nerve.

5. Zulinqi (GB 41)

Location: In the depression distal to the junction of the fourth and fifth metatarsal bones, on the lateral side of the tendon of m. extensor digiti minimi of the foot. (See Fig. 46)

Method: The patient sits. Press the point in the direction of the fifth metatarsal bone.

Reactions: Local soreness, numbness, distension conducted upward to the legs; warm sensation over the whole body.

Indications: Paralysis of the lower limbs and headache.

*Regional anatomy*

Vasculature: The dorsal arterial and venous network of the foot, the fourth dorsal metatarsal artery and vein.

Innervation: The branch of the intermediate dorsal cutaneous nerve of the foot.

6. Chengfu (BL 36)

Location: In the middle of the transverse gluteal fold. Locate the point with the patient in a prone position. (See Figs. 47 & 48)

Method: Press or press and knead the point.

Reactions: Local soreness, distension, numbness conducted to the foot.

Indications: Pain in the lower back and leg, fecal and urinal incontinence, pain, numbness and motor impairment of the lower extremities.

*Regional anatomy*

Vasculature: The artery and vein running alongside the sciatic nerve.

Innervation: The posterior femoral cutaneous nerve; deeper, the sciatic nerve.

7. Yinmen (BL 37)

Location: 6 *cun* below Chengfu (BL 36) on the line joining Chengfu (BL 36) and Weizhong (BL 40). (See Figs. 47 & 48)

Method: The patient lies in prone position or stands up. Press or press and knead the point.

Reactions: Local soreness, distension.

Indications: Pain in the lower back and thigh, numbness and motor impairment

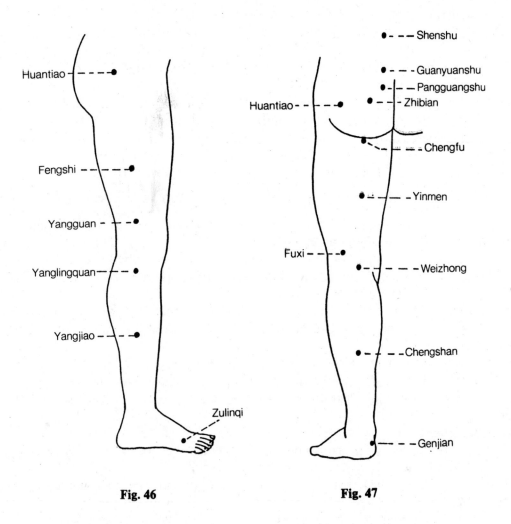

**Fig. 46**        **Fig. 47**

of the lower extremities, hemiplegia.

*Regional anatomy*

Vasculature: Laterally, the third perforating branches of the deep femoral artery and vein.

Innervation: The posterior femoral cutaneous nerve; deeper, the sciatic nerve.

8. Fuxi (BL 38)

Location: One *cun* above Weizhong (BL 40) on the medial side of the tendon of m. biceps femoris. The point is located in a depression with the knee slightly flexed. (See Fig. 47)

Method: Percuss, press or press and knead the point.

Reactions: Local soreness, distension, numbness conducted to the lateral side of the foot.

Indications: Paralysis of the lower extremities, pain in the knee joint.

*Regional anatomy*

Vasculature: The superolateral genicular artery and vein.

Innervation: The posterior femoral cutaneous nerve and the common peroneal nerve.

Muscles: Between musculi biceps femoris and vastus lateralis.

9. Weizhong (BL 40)

Location: Midpoint of the transverse crease of the popliteal fossa, between the tendons of m. biceps femoris and m. semitendinosus. (See Figs. 47 & 48)

Method: Percuss, press or press and knead the point.

Reactions: Local soreness, distension, numbness conducted to the foot.

Indications: Ischialgia, pain in the knee joints, motor impairment of the lower extremities.

*Regional anatomy*

Vasculature: Superficially, the femoropopliteal vein; deeper and medially, the popliteal vein; deepest, the popliteal artery.

Innervation: The posterior femoral cutaneous nerve, the tibial nerve.

Muscle: Between the caputs lateral and medial m. gastrocnemii.

10. Chengshan (BL 57)

Location: Directly below the belly of m. gastrocnemius, on the line joining Weizhong (BL 40) and tendo calcaneus, about 8 *cun* below Weizhong (BL 40). (See Figs. 47 & 48)

Method: The patient lies prone. Percuss, press or press and knead the point.

Reactions: Local soreness, distension conducted to the sole of the foot.

Indications: Ischialgia, paralysis of the lower limbs, pain in the lumbar region, constipation.

*Regional anatomy*

Vasculature: The small saphenous vein; deeper, the posterior tibial artery and vein.

Innervation: The medial sural cutaneous nerve; deeper, the tibial nerve.

11. Genjian

Location: Midpoint of tuber calcanei.

Method: Percuss or press the point.

Reactions: Local pain, distension conducted to the sole of the foot. (See Fig. 47)

Indications: Pain in calcaneus, paralysis of the lower limbs, infantile indigestion.

*Regional anatomy*

Vasculature: The medial calcaneus branches of the posterior tibial artery.

Innervation: The medial calcaneus cutaneous branches of the tibial nerve.

12. Jimai (LR 12)

Location: Inferior and lateral to the pubic spine, 2.5 *cun* lateral to the Ren Meridian, at the inguinal groove. (See Figs. 49 & 52)

Method: The patient lies in supine position. Press or press and knead the point.

Reactions: Local soreness, warmth, distension, numbness conducted to the knee and foot.

Indications: Paralysis of the lower limbs, fecal and urinal incontinence, enuresis.

*Regional anatomy*

Vasculature: The branches of the external pudendal artery and vein, the pubic branches of the inferior epigastric artery and vein; laterally, the femoral vein.

Innervation: The ilioinguinal nerve; deeper, in the inferior aspect, the anterior branch of the obturator nerve.

13. Biguan (ST 31)

Location: At the crossing point of intertsection between the line drawn directly down from the anterior superior iliac spine and the line level with the lower border of the symphysis pubis, in the depression on the lateral side of m. sartorius when the thigh is flexed. (See Fig. 49)

Method: Percuss, press or press and knead the point.

Reactions: Local soreness, distension, numbness conducted to the knee joint.

Indications: Pain in the knee joint, motor impairment, numbness and pain of the lower extremities.

*Regional anatomy*

Vasculature: Deeper, the branches of the lateral circumflex femoral artery and vein.

Innervation: The lateral femoral cutaneous nerve.

Muscles: M. sartorius, m. tensor fascial latal.

14. Futu (ST 32)

Location: On the line connecting the anterior superior iliac spine and lateral border of the patella, 6 *cun* above the laterosuperior border of the patella, in musculus rectus femoris. (See Fig. 49)

Method and Reactions: See Biguan (ST 31).

Indications: Pain in the knee, paralysis or motor impairment and pain of the lower extremities.

*Regional anatomy*

Vasculature: The branches of the lateral circumflex femoral artery and vein.

Innervation: The anterior and lateral femoral cutaneous nerves.

15. Zusanli (ST 36)

Location: One finger-breadth from the anterior crest of the tibia, in m. tibialis anterior. (See Fig. 50)

Method: Percuss, press or press and knead the point.

Reactions: Local soreness, numbness conducted to the tip of the toes.

Indications: Paralysis of the lower limbs, gastric pain, diarrhoea, dysentery, pain in the knee joint.

*Regional anatomy*

Vasculature: The anterior tibial artery and vein.

Innervation: Superficially, the lateral sural cutaneous nerve and the cutaneous branch of the saphenous nerve; deeper, the deep peroneal nerve.

Muscle: Upper portion of m. tibialis anterior.

16. Fenglong ( ST 40)

Location: 8 *cun* superior and anterior to the external malleolus, about one finger-breadth posterior to Tiaokou (ST 38). (See Fig. 50)

Method: The patient sits upright or lies supine. Percuss or press the point.

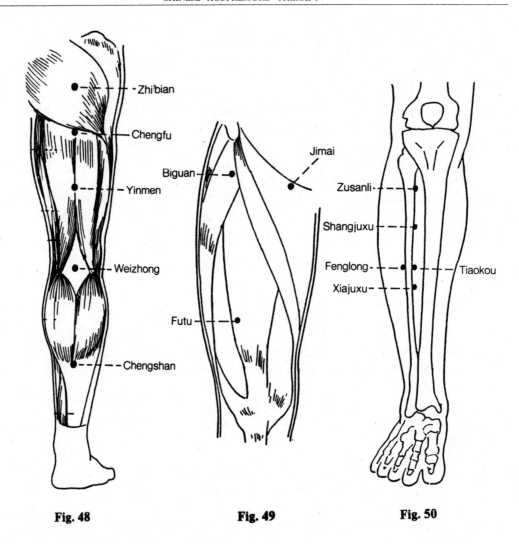

**Fig. 48**                          **Fig. 49**                          **Fig. 50**

Reactions: Local distension, numbness.

Indications: Numbness or pain in the cerural region, motor impairment, pain, swelling or paralysis of the lower extremities.

*Regional anatomy*

Vasculature: The branches of the anterior tibial artery and vein.

Innervation: The superficial peroneal nerve.

Muscle: The lateral border of venter of m. tibialis anterior.

17. Heding (EX-LE 2)

Location: Above the knee, in the depression at the midpoint of the upper border of the patella. (See Fig. 51)

Method: The patient sits upright or lies supine. Percuss, press or press and knead the point.

Reactions: Soreness, distension in the knee.

Indications: Knee pain, weakness of the foot and leg, paralysis of the lower limbs.

*Regional anatomy*

Vasculature: Network of the arteries around the knee joint formed by the branches of the profunda fermoris artery, fermoris artery and branches of the anterior, posterior tibial arteries.

Innervation: The anterior femoral cutaneous nerve.

18. Jiexi (ST 41)

Location: At the midpoint of the transverse crease of the ankle joint, in the depression between the tendons of m. extensor digitorum longus and hallucis longus, approximately at the level of the tip of the external malleolus. (See Fig. 51)

Method: Press the point.

Reactions: Local soreness, numbness, distension conducted to the dorsum and tips of the toes.

Indications: Pain in the ankle joint, pain and paralysis of the lower extremities, epilepsy, headache.

*Regional anatomy*

Vasculature: The anterior tibial artery and vein.

Innervation: The superficial and deep peroneal nerve.

19. Jimen (SP 11)

Location: At the middle lower 1/3 anterior aspect of the thigh, and medial border of musculus sartorius. (See Fig. 52)

Method: Press or press and knead the point.

Reactions: Local soreness, distension conducted to the medial side of the knee joint.

Indications: Urinary blockage, enuresis, swelling and pain in the inguinal region.

*Regional anatomy*

Vasculature: Superficially, the great saphenous vein; deeper on the lateral side, the femoral artery and vein.

Innervation: The anterior femoral cutaneous nerve; deeper, the saphenous nerve.

Muscles: Musculi sartorius, adductor longus, adductor magnus.

20. Yinlingquan (SP 9)

Location: On the lower border of the medial condyle of the tibia, in the depression between the posterior border of the tibia and m. gastrocnemius. (See Fig. 52)

Method: The patient sits upright or lies supine. Press, percuss or press and knead the point.

Reactions: Local soreness, distension conducted to the foot.

Indications: Paralysis of the lower limbs, abdominal pain and distension, diarrhoea, dysentery, urinary incontinence, irregular menstruation, pain in the knee.

*Regional anatomy*

Vasculature: In an anterior position, the great saphenous vein, the genu suprema artery; deeper, the posterior tibial artery and vein.

Innervation: Superficially, the medial crural cutaneous nerve; deeper, the tibial nerve.

Muscle: Anterior border of caput medial m. gastrocnemius.

21. Lougu (SP 7)

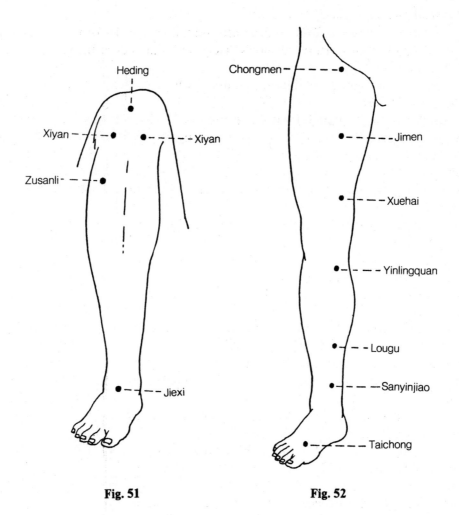

Heding

Xiyan — Xiyan

Zusanli

Jiexi

Chongmen

Jimen

Xuehai

Yinlingquan

Lougu

Sanyinjiao

Taichong

**Fig. 51**          **Fig. 52**

Location: 3 *cun* above Sanyinjiao (SP 6), on the line joining the tip of the medial malleolus and Yinlingquan (SP 9). (See Fig. 52)

Method: Percuss, press or press and knead the point.

Reactions: Local soreness, distension, numbness conducted to the posterior aspect of the leg and the sole of the foot.

Indications: Abdominal distension, borborygmus, coldness and numbness of the knees and legs, paralysis of the lower limbs.

*Regional anatomy*

Vasculature: The great saphenous vein, the posterior tibial artery and vein.

Innervation: Superficially, the medial crural cutaneous nerve; deeper, in the posterior aspect, the tibial nerve.

22. Sanyinjiao (SP 6)

Location: 3 *cun* directly above the tip of the medial malleolus, on the posterior border of the medial aspect of the tibia. (See Fig. 52)

Method: Percuss, press or press and knead the point.

Reactions: Local soreness, distension, conducted to the medial side of the foot.

Indications: Abdominal pain, borborygmus, abdominal distension, diarrhoea, disorder in the reproductive system, headache, dizziness and vertigo, insomnia.

*Regional anatomy* See Lougu (SP 7).

23. Taichong (LR 3)

Location: On the dorsum of the foot, in the depression distal to the junction of the first and second metatarsal bones. (See Fig. 52)

Method: The patient sits. Press on the point in the direction of the first metatarsal bone.

Reactions: Local soreness, numbness, distension conducted upward to the legs or warm sensation over the whole body.

Indications: Headache, dizziness and vertigo, paralysis of the lower limbs.

*Regional anatomy*

Vasculature: The dorsal venous network of the foot, the first dorsal metatarsal artery.

Innervation: The branch of the superficial peroneal nerve, cutaneous dorsal medial nerve.

24. Zhiguanjie

Location: At the transverse creases of the proximal and distal interphalangeal joints of the digiti planta pedis. (See Fig. 53)

Method: The patient takes any convenient position. Poke the points with the fingernail.

Reactions: Local pain, warmth; in some cases, there is a sensation of warmth and distension in the head.

Indications: Paralysis of the lower extremities, shock, dizziness.

*Regional anatomy*

Vasculature: Digital plantar arteries and veins.

Innervation: Digital plantar nerves.

25. Zhijiagen

Location: On the five toenail folds. (See Fig. 53)

Method: The patient takes a convenient position. Poke the points with the fingernail.

Reactions: Local pain and warmth; in some cases, the feeling of warmth and distension spreads to the head.

Indications: Paralysis of the lower extremities, shock, dizziness.

*Regional anatomy*: See Zhiguanjie.

26. Yongquan (KI 1)

Location: On the sole, in the depression when the foot is in plantar flexion, approximately at the junction of the anterior third and posterior two-thirds of the sole. (See Fig. 54)

Method: The patient lies supine or prone. Percuss, press or press and knead the point.

Reactions: Local soreness, distension, pain.

Indications: Infantile convulsions, loss of consciousness, headache, dizziness,

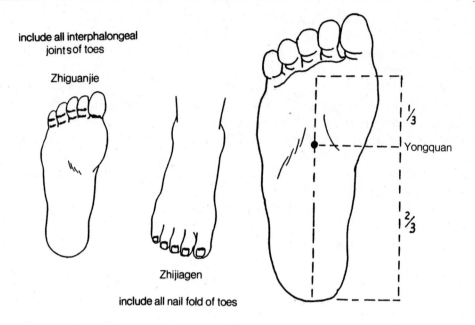

include all interphalongeal joints of toes

Zhiguanjie

Zhijiagen

include all nail fold of toes

$\frac{1}{3}$

Yongquan

$\frac{2}{3}$

**Fig. 53**                                      **Fig. 54**

sunstroke, paralysis of the lower limbs.

*Regional anatomy*

Vasculature: Deeper, the plantar arterial arch.

Innervation: The second common plantar digital nerve.

Muscles: Musculi flexor digitorum brevis, oponeurosis plantaris.

## C. Stimulation-Lines

There are sixteen stimulaton-lines distributed over the surface of the body.

### 1. Stimulation-lines on the upper extremities

*The first line*: Starting from the radial end of the transverse crease of the palmar aspect of the wrist, it goes upward along the radial side of the forearm, through the prominence of m. brachoradialis, stopping at the radial end of the elbow transverse crease. It corresponds to a part of the Lung Meridian of Hand-Taiyin. (See Fig. 55)

*The second line:* Starting from the midpoint of the transverse crease of the palmar aspect of the wrist, it goes upward along the middle line of the forearm, passing through the elbow joint, and then upward along the m. biceps brachii, stopping at the anterior portion of the shoulder joint. It corresponds to a part of the Pericardium Meridian of Hand-Jueyin. (See Fig. 55)

*The third line:* Starting from the ulnar end of the transverse crease of the palmar aspect of the wrist, it goes upward along the ulnar side of the forearm, passing through the medial side of the elbow joint and upper arm, stopping at the anterior end of the axillary crease. It corresponds to a part of the Heart Meridian of Hand-Shaoyin. (See Fig. 55)

*The fourth line*: Starting from the ulnar end of the dorsal transverse crease of the wrist, it goes upward along the ulnar side of the forearm, passing through the medial side of the elbow joint and upper arm, stopping at the posterior end of the axillary crease. It corresponds to a part of the Small Intestine Meridian of Hand-Taiyang. (See Fig. 56)

*The fifth line*: Starting from the dorsal aspect of second, third, fourth, and fifth metacarpal phalangeal joints, it goes upward along the tendon of m. extensor digitorum, comes together with it at the midpoint of the dorsal aspect of the wrist, and passes along the midline of the dorsal aspect of the forearm, stopping at the posterior part of the elbow joint. It corresponds to a part of the Sanjiao Meridian of Hand-Shaoyang. (See Fig. 56)

*The sixth line*: Starting from the radial end of the transverse crease dorsal aspect of the wrist, it goes upward along the radial side of the forearm, passing through the lateral side of the elbow joint and then along the space between m. biceps brachii and m. triceps brachii, stopping at the acromion. It corresponds to a part of the Large Intestine Meridian of Hand-Yangming. (See Fig. 56)

### 2. Stimulation-lines on the back and lumbar regions

*The first line*: Starting from the posterior hairline of the neck, it goes downward along either side of the spinal column at 5 cm lateral, stopping at either side of the lumbosacral joint. It corresponds to a part of the first line of the Bladder Meridian of Foot-Taiyang. (See Fig. 56)

*The second line*: Starting from either side of the first thoracic vertebra, 8 cm lateral to the spinal column, it passes downward and stops at the upper border of the sacral bone. It corresponds to a part of the second line of the Bladder Meridian of Foot-Taiyang on the back. (See Fig. 56)

### 3. Stimulation-lines on the lower extremities

*The first line*: Starting from the anterior portion of the ankle joint, it goes upward along the m. tibialis anterior, passing through the lateral side of the patella and thigh, stopping at the posterior fossa of the spina iliaca anterior superior. It corresponds to a part of the Stomach Meridian of Foot-Yangming. (See Fig. 55)

*The second line*: Starting from the dorsal aspect of the five metatarsal phalangeal joints of the digiti pedis, it goes upward along each tendon of m. extensor digitorum longus to the anterior portion of the ankle joint, where the five tendons come together and pass through the lateral side of m. tibialis anterior, then passing upward through the lateral side of the knee joint and thigh and stopping at the spina iliaca anterior superior. It corresponds to a part of the Gall Bladder Meridian of Foot-Shaoyang. (See Fig. 55)

*The third line*: Starting from the medial side of the tendon calcaneus, it goes upward along the medial side of m. gastrocnemius, the knee joint and m. gracilis, stopping at the insertion of m. gracilis. It corresponds to a part of the Kidney Meridian of Foot-Shaoyin. (Fig. 57)

*The fourth line*: Starting from the posterior fossa of malleolus medialis, it goes upward along the space between m. tibia and m. gastrocnemius, passing through the medial side of the knee joint. It is divided into two branches: one of them going along

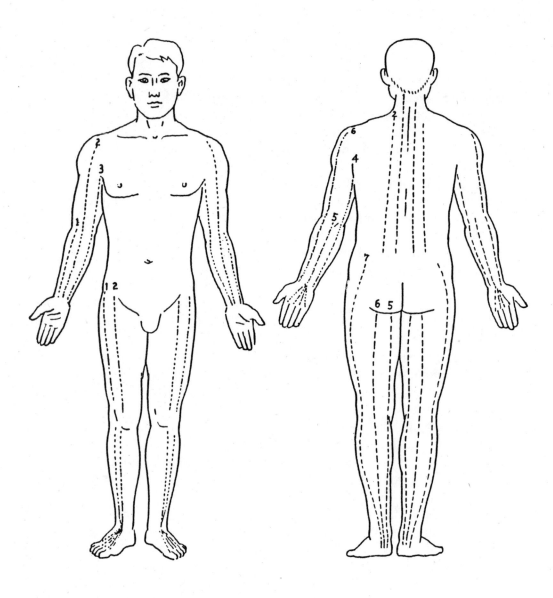

Fig. 55   Stimulation lines for
acupressure therapy (anterior)

Fig. 56   Stimulation lines for
acupressure therapy (posterior)

the prominence of m. sartorius and stopping at spina iliaca anterior superior; the other branch going along the prominence of m. adductor magnus and stopping at the inguen.

It corresponds to a part of the Liver Meridian of Foot-Jueyin and the Spleen Meridian of Foot-Taiyin. (See Fig. 57)

*The fifth line*: Starting from the insertion of tendon calcaneus, it goes upward along the prominence of m. gastrocnemius, passing through the medial end of the popliteal transverse crease, upward along the space of m. semimembranous and m. biceps femoris, stopping at the tuber ischiadium. It corresponds to a part of the Bladder Meridian of Foot-Taiyang. (Fig. 56)

*The sixth line:* Starting from the midpoint of the insertion of tendon calcaneus, it goes upward along the middle line of m. gastrocnemius, passing through the popliteal fossa and the space between m. semitendonoxus, m. semimembranoxus and m. biceps femoris, stopping at the tuber ischiadium. It corresponds to a part of the Bladder Meridian of Foot-Taiyang. (See Fig. 56)

*The seventh line*: Starting from malleolus lateralis, it goes upward along the lateral prominence of m. gastrocnemius and the lateral end of the popliteal transverse crease, passing through the prominence of m. biceps femoris, and the major trochanter,

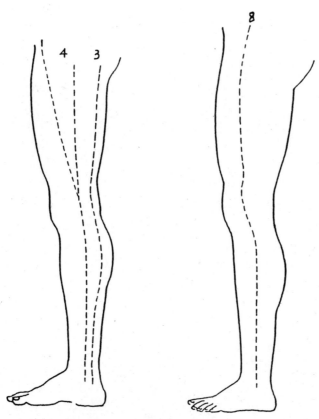

**Fig. 57   Lower extremities for**
**acupressure therapy (internal and external)**

stopping at the lateral side of spina iliaca posterior superior. (See Fig. 56)

*The eighth line*: Starting from mallealus lateralis, it goes upward along the prominence of m. peroneus longus to the anterior portion of caput fibula, passing upward through the lateral side of the patella and the lateral border of m. vastus lateralis, stoppping at the midpoint of crista iliaca. It corresponds to a part of the Gall Bladder Meridian of Foot-Shaoyang. (See Fig. 57)

# Chapter Two
## Clinical Study

### Section I
### Diseases of the Nervous System

#### A. Sequelae of Cerebral Birth Injury

The term refers to direct or indirect injuries of the infant's intracranial tissues and the corresponding symptoms that occur during delivery. Causatively, the injuries are of two types:

1. Mechanical injury. The fetus' cranial bone is thin and elastic. The fibrous membrane connecting individual bones has some degree of plasticity to facilitate passage through the birth canal. However, excessive compression during parturition may deform the infant's head, leading to intracranial injury. Congestion in the birth canal may be caused by a number of factors, such as breech presentation, induced labour after breech presentation, use of high forceps, overly long or short parturition time, narrow or deformed pelvis, oversized infant's head, amongst others. Such injuries occur more frequently in cases of premature delivery or first birth.

2. Anoxic injury. In the course of delivery, any factor that hinders the normal supply of oxygen to the fetus may result in anoxic brain damage. Although neonates are much less vulnerable to anoxia than adults, a severe lack of oxygen will increase blood vessel penetration and lead to spotted cerebral hemorrhage, cerebral edema and blood stasis. Severe anoxia is often caused by stagnant delivery due to weak uterine contraction, prepartal bleeding, high fever, intoxication during pregnancy, abruption placentae, inhalation of amnionic fluid, blood circulatory obstruction, oppression of the chest and asphyxia caused by other factors.

*Classification of cerebral birth injury*

1. Laceration of dural septum, mainly that of the falx of the cerebrum; and tentorium of the cerebellum. (See Fig. 58)

2. Intracranial hemorrhage or hematoma. Epidural hematoma is rarely seen, while infradural hematoma is one of the most common causes of death in infants. Subarachnoid hematoma is mostly found in premature infants, occurring mostly in the fourth or side chamber. There are also multiple hemorrhages of mixed types. (see Fig. 59)

3. Hemorrhage of a substantial part of the brain. This is rarely caused by simple instrumental injury which is often local. However, macular extravasation of a substantial part of the brain and extensive blood stasis on the pia mater may appear if the injury is associated with severe anoxic lesions.

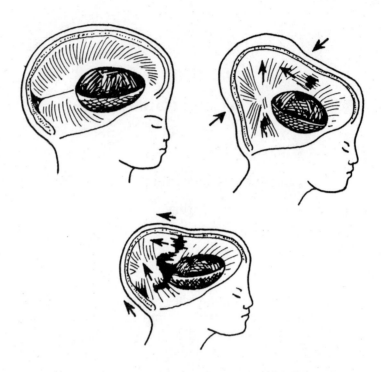

Fig. 58    Laceration of falx of cerebrum and tentorium of
cerebelli in neonate due to skull deformation

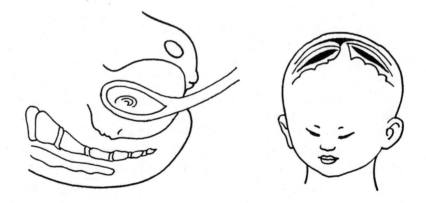

Fig. 59    Intracranial hemorrhage occurring during parturition

It should be pointed out that the causes of partal injuries are often both mechanical and anemic/anoxic. In some cases, the two causes cannot be identified separately. According to the 150 cases of cerebral birth injuries studied in the Institute of Orthopedics and Traumatology, the causes are as follows:

(a) Anoxic stagnant delivery, 62 cases (41%);

(b) Anoxic and instrumental injury, 39 cases (26%);

(c) Improper midwifery manipulation, 16 cases (11%);

(d) Caesarean operation owing to anoxia, 11 cases (8%);

(e) Anemia and anoxia due to umbilical tangling round the neck, 10 cases (6%);

(f) Induced delivery after breech presentation, 8 cases (5%);

(g) Hemorrhage due to early exfoliation of placenta, 4 cases (3%).

*Symptoms:*

The neonates' clinical symptoms are complicated, such as asphyxia, dyspnea or irregular respiration accompanied by pallor or cyanosis, weak or sharp cry, trembling, low body temperature, vomiting, fast or slow pulsation. Although the locus and degree of the injuries differ, the common clinical manifestations are: rigid paralysis, increased muscle tension, hyperactive tendon reflexes, diminishment or loss of superficial skin reflexes, pathological reflexes such as Babinski's Sign, Hoffmann's Sign, patella and ankle clonus being positive. There is no muscle atrophy.

Severe cases show mental retardation, dysphasia, salivation and fecal and urinary incontinence. There is also muscle spasm of the extremities which affects functional activities. The arm is bent close to the chest and the elbow is flexed, accompanied by limited supination of the forearm, drop wrist, inharmonious finger movements, complete or partial loss of hand functions and walking with stiffened limbs. The adductor group of the thigh muscles are spasmodic due to spasm of musculi biceps, semitendinous, semimembraneous, gastrocnemius and soleus, resulting in knock-knee, taut foot, talipes equinovarus and walking in limping or dragging steps. Some patients have rigid neck, opisthognathous, general or localized epilepsy.

*Treatment*

Diagnostic differentiation: On the basis of case history and clinical manifestations, these expressions are the results of deficiency of the vital function and vital essence of the kidney, and insufficiency of the brain and closed apertures. According to the traditional Chinese medicine, these are attributed to spasm of the muscles along the channels, especially in the limbs, and five weaknesses and five stagnations. Therefore, the treatment should be aimed at reinforcing the kidney, invigorating the functions of the brain, activating blood circulation, opening the apertures and relieving spasm.

Method: Use the regular acupressure techniques for treating paralysis, such as manipulation routine, selection of points and stimulation-lines. Supplementary orthopedic manipulations and methods are also used.

*Commonly used points for treating paralysis:*

1. Points on the head and neck: Baihui (DU 20), Shuaigu (GB 8), Tianzhu (BL 10), Fengchi (GB 20), Wangu (GB 12), Yamen (DU 15), Dazhui (GB 14).

2. Points on the upper extremities: Jianyu (LI 15), Binao (LI 14), Naohui (SJ 13), Zhima, Jihui, Ximen (PC 4), Yangchi (SJ 4), Yangxi (LI 5), Zhangjian, Hegu (LI 4),

Zhiguanjie, Zhijiagen.

3. Points on the lower extremities: Huantiao (GB 30), Futu (LI 18), Fengshi (GB 31), Jimen (SP 11), Fuxi (BL 38), Weizhong (BL 40), Chengshan (BL 57), Lougu (SP 7), Yangjiao (GB 35), Genjian, Taichong (LR 3), Zulinqi (GB 41), Zhiguanjie, Zhijiagen, etc.

4. Points on the lower back: Yaoyan (EX-B 7), Guanyuanshu (BL 26), etc.

*Points for treating salivation, dysphasia, and difficulty in swallowing:* Yingxiang (LI 20), Jiachengjiang (Extra), Chengjiang (RN 24), Lianquan (RN 23), Shanglianquan (Extra), Chuigen, and Dicang (ST 4). For manipulations, see Figs 60, 61, 62, 63, 64, and 65.

*Commonly used stimulation-lines for treating paralysis:* The second, third, fifth and sixth are the main lines in the upper extremities; while in the lower extremities, the main lines are the first, second, fourth, fifth and seventh. Also the sector of the Du Meridian in the neck, chest and lumbar regions.

Course of treatment: A complete course consists of 15-20 treatments given once every day or every other day. The courses may be repeated once or twice.

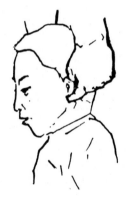

**Fig. 60    Pressing Chuigen point**

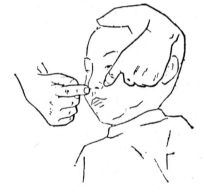

**Fig. 61    Pressing Yingxiang point**

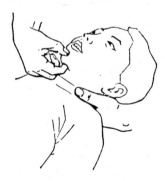

**Fig. 62    Pressing Chengjiang
and Lianquan points**

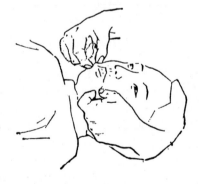

**Fig. 63    Pinching orbicularis oris muscle**

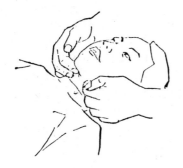

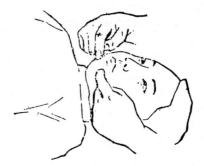

**Fig. 64   Pressing Jiachengjiang point**

**Fig. 65   Massaging along submandibular region**

Response: Light perspiration indicates right effect.

*Commonly used orthopedic manipulations in the treatment of paralysis:*

1. Orthotherapy for supination disability of the forearm. (See Fig. 13)

2. Manipulation for tendons of the fingers to relax the flexion contracture of the fingers. (See Fig. 14)

3. Method of separating the hip (frog-type test) to relieve the spasm of the adduction muscles of the hip. (See Fig. 15)

4. Raising the stretched lower extremity, supplemented by massage with three fingers to relieve the spasm of the posterior muscle group of the thigh. (See Fig. 16)

5. Internal and external rotation of the hip (head of femur) to remove disturbance; internal and external rotation of the thigh. (See Figs. 17 & 18)

6. Orthopedic manipulation of 4-form type in prone position to relieve the spasm of the muscles of the iliac, waist regions and rectus femoris. (See Fig. 19)

7. Manipulation of the iliotibial tract to relieve the spasm of the tract. (See Fig. 20)

8. Treating drop-foot by pressing the knee. (See Fig. 21)

9. Massage the posterior aspect of the leg with three fingers while flexing the knee to 90° and pressing the sole to treat drop-foot. (See Fig. 22)

10. Pushing and pulling the foot to treat strephexpodia and strophexopodia. (See Fig. 23)

11. Pressing the foot to treat claw-foot. (See Fig. 24)

Along with these orthopedic operations, the spasmodic muscles should be pressed and massaged at the corresponding points or along the stimulation-lines. The operations should be performed step by step, gently and steadily. Forceful violent operations do not help speed up the healing process, but will instead exacerbate the injury.

## B. Sequelae of Cerebral Trauma

Brain trauma is a common injury, accounting for about 20 percent of all bodily injuries in either war or peace time; its incidence ranking next only to that of injuries of the extremities. However, the mortality rate seems to be the highest of that for all traumas. Mild cases, if given timely treatment, may recover completely. However, some of these cases are followed by sequelae in varying degrees and need further treatment.

*Symptoms*

Some patients suffering from sequelae of cerebral injury may experience dementia, headache, dizziness, tinnitus, poor vision or even loss of eyesight, hemiplegia, dysphasia, aphasia and epilepsy. More frequently, such patients experience multiple complaints over a long period of time, but neurological examinations show no irregularities. The "sequelae of brain trauma" discussed here refer to symptoms which appear shortly after cerebral trauma and persist after more than three months of treatment, and to cases where examinations of the nervous system produce no positive findings.

*Locational diagnosis*

Central paralysis caused by trauma of the pyramidal tract. The locality of the injuries varies. (See Fig. 66)

1. Lesion in the motor area of the cerebral cortex of gyrus precentralis may develop contralateral paralysis of an arm or a leg. It may also be associated with motor aphasia and localized epilepsy (Jacksonian epilepsy).

2. Lesion in the internal capsule may produce contralateral hemiplegia, in which case the upper extremity is worse than the lower, the distal part is worse than the proximal part and the lower facial muscle and half of the tongue muscle on the paralyzed side are also paralytic. Other muscles controlled by cranial nerves and trunk muscles, however, do not manifest paralysis, as these muscles are controlled by hemispheric nerves on either side. The posterior part of the internal capsule of the pyramidal tract has a sense tract and a sight fiber going through it. If this is involved, there will be an increased hemiparesthesia and hemiopia.

3. Brain stem trauma (midbrain, pons, medulla oblongata) will lead to contralateral cerebral hemiplegia and peripheral cranial nerve paralysis on the same side. If the injury involves the medial lemniscus and spinal lemniscus, such cross paralysis may also be accompanied by hemianesthesia on the paralytic side of the body.

4. In the case of spinal cord trauma, complete transverse injuries above the cervical enlargement will produce quadriplegia, and those between the cervical and the lumbar enlargements will result in paraplegia, both accompanied by conductive tract hypoesthesia below the plane of the injuries, and impairment of bowel movement and urination. Partial transverse damage to the spinal cord on the side will produce Brown-Sequard's syndrome of centroparalysis and the loss of deep sensation on the same side as the damage, as well as the loss of dermatalgic and thermesthesic sensation on the contralateral side of the trunk.

*Diagnosis*

A clear case of early brain trauma accompanied by the above-mentioned symptoms and signs. Clear differentiation is necessary between post-traumatic organic pathologicl changes and the sequelae of cerebral damage.

*Treatment*

1. Acupressure therapy. See therapeutic measures listed for treatment of paralysis and cerebral birth injury.

2. Orthopedic therapy. See therapeutic methods listed for treatment of sequelae of

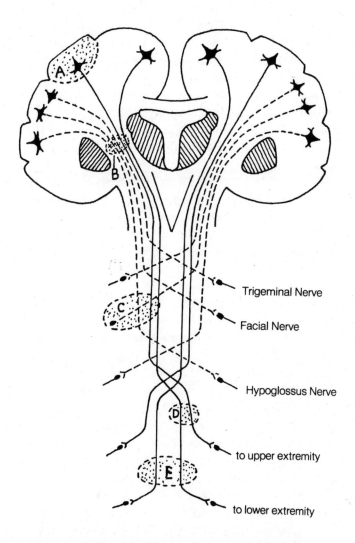

**Fig. 66  Diagram of lesions of the pyramidal tract**
**a. Lesion in motor area of cerebral cortex of gyrus precentralis**
**b. Lesion in capsula interna**
**c. Lesion in one side of pons**
**d. Lesion in one side of cervical segment of vertebral column**
**e. Transverse lesion of thoracic segment of vertebral column**

cerebral birth injury.

*Case report*

Case 1: Lin, male, aged 36, an electrician, case history No. 22213.

His first visit was on April 11, 1984 when he complained of having been knocked down by a car three years before, and had since suffered from headache, dysphasia, loss of body balance and dysfunction of extremities. He came to the outpatient department supported by two persons.

Examination findings: Consciousness unaffected, alalia with vocal difficulty, hypertonicity of both upper and lower extremities; hyperactive tendon reflexes and diminished superficial reflexes. Pathological reflexes such as Hoffmann's sign and Babinski's sign were positive, patella and ankle clonus positive, no muscular atrophy. Prior to acupressure treatment, examination by somatosensory electrically evoked potential showed that the stimulation-site was the median nerve on the left wrist, and the record-site was at the hand sensation region on the right cerebral cortex. The latent period was obviously prolonged to over 40 ms°.

After acupressure therapy on the four extremities, the trunk, the head and the neck once every other day, (see "sequelae of cerebral birth injury" for manipulation details), there was marked improvement. After forty treatments, the above symptoms disappeared.

Case 2: Ma, male, aged six, case history No. 24312.

His first visit was on July 2, 1984. The patient had fallen from the second floor about six months before, resulting in a comminuted compression fracture of the right parietal bone complicated by hematoma in the epidural space, and laceration of the cerebral cortex tissue in the right temple region. Four days after the injury, drainage of the hematoma in the right epidural space was performed. However, dysfunction of the left arm and leg followed the operation. The left forearm showed difficulty in supination, muscular contraction on flexion of the fingers and drop-wrist. The left hand was unable to hold objects. He walked unsteadily, with a limping left leg, dragging steps and the toes kicking the ground. He had spastic contracture of musculus biceps femoris and the semimembranous and semitendonous muscles behind the left thigh, of the adductor muscle group of the left thigh and of musculi gastrocnemius and saleus, resulting in equinovarus deformity. Having been treated about sixty times, the patient recovered. Examination after the last treatment on November 22, 1984, showed general restoration of the left hand functions and release of the contracted muscles of the left lower extremity. The left equinovarus deformity was almost completely corrected, leaving only a slight limp.

Case 3. Zhao, male, aged 40, case history No. 24621, an administrator.

His first visit was on July 21, 1984. Complaints: headache, dizziness, nausea, vomiting, tinnitus, poor vision and memory, numbness and tiredness. He mentioned having been knocked over by a car and injuring his left frontal bone with intracranial hemorrhage. Six months earlier, he had had an emergency operation to clear the hematoma in the skull.

Prior to treatment in our clinic, his electroencephalogram, somatosensory-evoked potential test and electromyogram showed nothing abnormal. It was diagnosed as sequelae of brain trauma. Acupressure manipulation on the head, neck, back and the right upper and lower extremities was performed. The selected points and stimulation-lines and the manipulation routine were similar to those selected for sequelae of cerebral birth injury. After forty treatments, the above symptoms disappeared.

## C. Sequelae of Cervical Spinal Cord Injury

Injury of the spinal cord frequently occurs during war or peace time. It is a serious injury often resulting in disability or death.

*Types of Injury*

Causatively, spinal cord injury is of two kinds, closed and open. The open type occurs mostly in war-time as a result of wounds caused by sharp edges or firearms, whilst the closed type occurs mostly during peace time, as a result of violent blows to the spine. The types commonly seen are as follows:

1. When the direction of the blow causes the spinal column to be overflexed so that the pyramides squeeze and extrude heavily on one another, causing compressive fracture of the pyramides, with the intervertebral discs herniating backward and compressing the spinal cord or the nerve roots.

2. When the direction of the blow causes the spinal column to become over-stretched and the subflavous ligament to crease and protrude into the vertebral canal so that the spinal cord is crushed and damaged.

3. When the direction of the blow is nearly vertical to the spinal column, causing dislocation of the vertebrae, rupture of the anterior and posterior longitudinal ligaments, fracture of the articular process, depression of the vertebral plate, compression of the spinal cord or compression of the spinal cord between the dislocated vertebrae.

4. Spinal cord damage may occur in birth injury, especially during breech presentation. The force of traction experienced by the fetus bears mainly on the cervical vertebrae, which may lead to injury, sometimes even to laceration of the dura mater spinalis.

Any direct injury (such as that caused by bullets or shrapnel), or indirect injury (such as that caused by fractures in the spinal cord or compression resulting from dislocation) will result in complete and/or incomplete damage to the spinal cord.

*Symptoms*

1. Injury of the cervical segment of the spinal cord may lead to quadriplegia. The clinical manifestations of the lower extremities are attributable to upper motor neuron paralysis; those of the upper extremities are attributable to either upper or lower motor neuron paralysis, depending on the location of the injury. Sensational disturbance may involve the arm, neck, face and even the occipital region.

2. Injury of the upper neck (C1-3). The clinical manifestations may show muscle atrophy or paralysis of the neck and scapular suspensory in different degrees, spastic quadriplegia, increased muscle tone, hyperactive tendon reflexes, positive pathological reflexes, hiccups, vomiting, dyspnea, low voice or even complete respiratory paralysis. Nerve root pain occurs in the occipital region and posterior aspect of the neck, and it may also induce loss of sensation in these parts.

3. Middle segment (C4-6) injury of the cervical spinal cord. Manifestations:

quadriplegia, paralysis and muscle atrophy of musculi biceps brachi, supraspinatus, infraspinatus, subscapularis and teres minor—lower motor neuron paralysis; an increase of muscle tone and hyperactive reflex of m. triceps brachii, diminishment or loss of superficial sensation of the shoulder and scapular regions; decrease in or loss of skin sensation of the trunk below T2 level; loss of biceps brachial reflex but hyperactivity of triceps brachial reflex and tendon reflex of the lower extremities.

4. Injury of the lower neck segment (C7-8): Clinical manifestations: obvious paralysis of finger movements and atrophy of the small muscles of the hand; atrophy to varying degrees and flaccid paralysis of forearm muscles; nerve root pain confined to the forearm and hand; loss or diminution of segmental sensation in the upper extremities; trunk sensation ending at T2 level. The biceps brachial reflex remains normal but the triceps brachial reflex, radiaperiosteal reflex and finger flexion reflex vanish. Horner's syndrome occurs on the affected side.

*Treatment*

Principle of treatment: Strengthening the nerve by way of reinforcing the function of the brain, tonifying the tendon and bone and relaxing the spasm of the muscle.

*Methods*

1. Acupressure therapy: Follow routine for treating paralysis (see "sequelae of cerebral birth injury"). Dysfunction after cervical spinal cord injury may debilitate the upper and lower extremities. It is necessary to give generalized acupressure therapy, including the regions of the head and neck; the manipulations are usually intensive, but the intensity should vary with the health state, gender, age and tolerance of the patient. Manipulation should not be so strong as to cause bone fracture or injure internal organs, since the affected extremity has lost or diminished sensation.

Handle the injured parts carefully, select two or three sensitive points around the damaged area, and press and knead the points repeatedly until the area feels warm (incomplete paralysis).

Refer to earlier passages on sequelae of cerebral birth injury concerning fecal and urinal incontinence and bowel movement.

2. Other manipulations: When spinal injury is accompanied by fractures and soft tissue lesions, these must have healed before manipulations begin. For cases of cervical or lumbar vertebral injuries, rotate the neck or lumbar region in a sitting position. If there is slight dislocation of cervical or lumbar vertebrae, determine the direction of the dislocation and rotate the affected part in a fixed sitting position to achieve reduction of the dislocated vertebrae. For thoracic vertebral injuries, manipulative pressing of the affected area is administered with the patient in a prone position. These remedies often produce good results.

3. Supportive treatment: For cases with fractures or surgical fixtures, after the wound has healed, acupressure therapy combined with drugs and acupuncture may be given, following the routine for treating paralytic patients.

(a) Prevention of complications: Treatment should be given immediately to paralytic patients with complications such as bed-sores and infection of the lungs or urinary systems.

To prevent bed-sores, turn the patient over in bed frequently; massage the affected surface of the body with 50% alchohol solution; help the patient move the extremities; keep the body clean; the matress should be smooth and firm and cotton or air rings should be used under the sacrum, greater trochanter and heel. If bed-sores have already developed, free-skin graft or rotational skin flap graft may be performed. Healing plaster may also be used to facilitate recovery.

In order to prevent and treat infection of the urinary system in its early stage, the urinary bladder should not be allowed to overextend, nor should catheterization be used frequently. An in-dwelling catheter can be used under sterilized conditions and douched twice a day. At the same time acupressure therapy can be given to promote the recovery of the urinary bladder function.

To prevent and treat pulmonary infection, the patient must be helped to turn over in bed once every two hours and asked to breathe deeply and cough. Lift and spread his arms to do chest expansion exercises, or use clapping manipulation on the patient's chest wall to help prevent pulmonary infection.

Passive joint movements of the affected limbs with the help of the nurse should be kept up to prevent joint rigidity and deformities. The patient should also do exercises as much as possible, such as turning over in bed, sitting up, lifting the arms, clenching the fists, revolving the forearms, flexing and extending the lower extremities in a lateral recumbent position, stooping, crawling, stretching the leg all the way to the heel, standing with a support, walking on crutches, lifting the feet alternately whilst standing still, etc. Lumbar rotating exercises are recommended after a fracture has healed, and walking with crutches or a cane once the lower extremities are strong enough. Practise diphragmatic respiration lying supine, to activate the abdominal wall muscles. Exercise dorsal muscles in a prone position. After discharge from hospital, the patient should continue to do exercises with the help of his family so as to improve body functions.

*Prognosis*

For patients with spinal cord injury, give comprehensive treatment. Acupressure therapy often shows positive results, and it is applicable in either early or late stages. In general, if the injury is mild and recent, the treatment often produces more effective results than in severe and old cases. For transverse injuries of the spinal cord, acupressure therapy may play a useful role in promoting the passive movement of the joints, decreasing edema, improving blood circulation and preventing or curing muscular atrophy.

*Case report*

Case 1. Incomplete injury of cervical spinal cord.

Tang, male, 40 years old, case history No. A-716, an office worker.

His first visit dated on July 25, 1983. He complained of having been thrown off his bike by another cyclist. His head struck the ground and the fourth cervical vertebra was fractured and dislocated, resulting in incomplete paralysis of both arms and legs. He came to our clinic after a 6-week skull traction treatment in another hospital.

Examination showed upper and lower motor neuron damage. (See clinical manifestations of middle neck injury.) Symptoms and signs of upper motor neuron damage were found in both lower extremities.

Initial examinations showed that the fracture of the fourth cervical vertebra had healed; movements of all joints of the arms were limited but passive movement reached normal range. There was extensive muscle atrophy.

The left hand's gripping power was 4 kg, the right hand's zero, being unable to hold objects. Hoffmann's sign on both sides was positive. Both lower extremities showed extensive atrophy, with increased muscle tone. He was able to stand up and walk with the help of another person. The steps were unsteady and dragging. Babinski's sign showed positive on both sides. Excretion of urine and feces could not be controlled.

After 40 treatments with acupressure therapy, muscle atrophy of the four extremities recovered. The left hand's gripping power increased from 4 to 20 kg, whilst that of the right hand increased from zero to 10 kg.

Electromyogram of the median nerve and ulnar nerve showed that the pathological wave (thrilling, positive phase wave) had disappeared. (See Figs. 67, 68, 69, 70, 71, and 72)

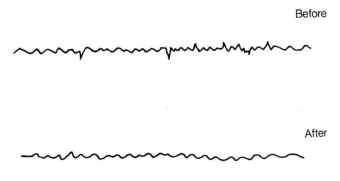

**Fig. 67    Eletromyogram results of relaxed short abductor muscle of right thumb before and after treatment**

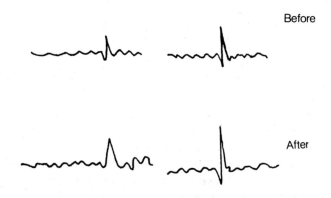

**Fig. 68    Electromyogram results of loosely contracted short abductor muscle of right thumb before and after treatment**

Before

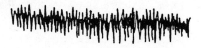

After

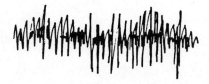

**Fig. 69    Electromyogram results of fully contracted short
abductor muscle of right thumb before and after treatment**

Before

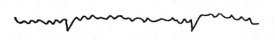

After

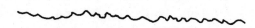

**Fig. 70    Electromyogram results of relaxed abductor
muscle of right small finger before and after treatment**

Control of urine and feces had returned to normal. Normal gait had been recovered for a distance of three kilometres without help. Hoffmann's sign showed positive on the left side, but that on the right side was negative; Babinski's sign was negative on both sides. Tang returned to his original job as a bus dispatcher.

Case 2. Incomplete cervical spinal cord injury.

Guo, male, 48 years old, case history No. 3013, an office worker.

He first visited our clinic on February 29, 1984 for treatment of incomplete high level paralysis due to traumatic dislocation between the 4th and 5th cervical vertebrae caused by a traffic accident three years before. Earlier, he had received skull traction treatment for six weeks and massage for three months in other hospitals. He was unable to walk without the help of another person. He could take care of urination and bowel

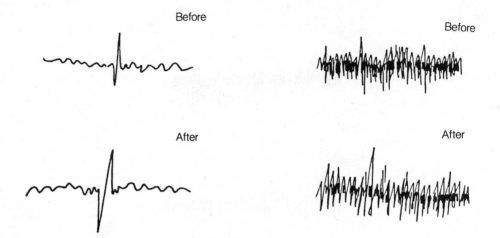

Before

After

Before

After

**Fig. 71   Electromyogram results of loosely contracted abductor muscle of right small finger before and after treatment**

**Fig. 72   Electromyogram results of fully contrated abductor muscle of right small finger before and after treatment**

movements by himself. However, his arms recovered rather slowly, especially the left arm.

Initial clinical findings: His general condition was good; active movements of the joints of both arms were limited, and passive movements could not reach normal range. No muscle atrophy. Skin sensation slightly diminished; deep reflexes hyperactive. Hoffmann's sign was positive on both sides. His left hand was unable to form a fist, the right hand's gripping power was 11 kg, but unsteady when holding objects, while the left hand was completely disabled.

He walked with a limp requiring the help of another person; the lower extremities showed no muscle atrophy; muscular power was 3-4 grade; skin sensation diminished; deep reflexes were hyperactive. Babinski's sign on both sides was positive. He was unable to look after himself.

Acupressure therapy: For the selection of the points and stimulation-lines on the head, neck, trunk, and four extremities, see section on acupressure treatment of sequelae of cerebral birth injury.

Treatment was given once every other day. After 80 treatments, the functions of the four extremities improved and he was able to look after himself. The results of re-examination by electromyogram and somatosensory evoked potential showed obvious progress. (See Figs. 73, 74, 75, and 76).

## D. Injury of the Thoracic Spinal Cord

Injury of the thoracic spinal cord may lead to spastic paralysis of both lower extremities. Abnormal dermal sensation was limited below the second thoracic vertebra and above the inguinal ligament. Main clinical manifestations were as follows: Spastic paralysis in the lower extremities and intercostal neuralgia; skin sensory disturbance above the second rib with the lesion located in T2; T4—above the nipple; T6—above

Before

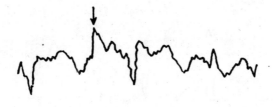

After

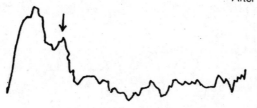

**Fig. 73    Results of examination of body-sensory evoked potential before and after treatment**

Before

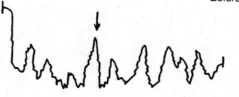

After

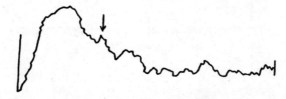

**Fig. 74    Results of examination of body-sensory evoked potential before and after treatment**

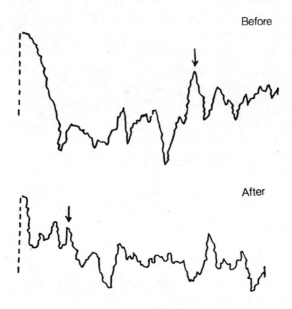

**Fig. 75    Results of examination of body-sensory evoked potential before and after treatment**

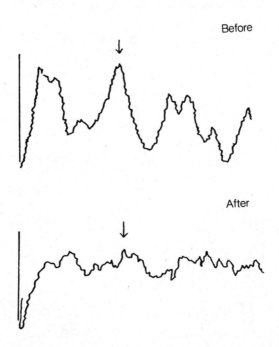

**Fig. 76    Results of examination of body-sensory evoked potential before and after treatment**

tip of xiphoid process; T8—above lower border of the rib; T10—the umbilicus; T12 —above the inguinal ligament. Tendon reflex of lower extremities showed hyperactivity when the lesion was located at T1-9, reflex was lost or diminished at the upper abdomen; T9-11, at middle abdomen; T11-L1, at lower abdomen.

*Case report*

Zheng, female, 35 years old, an accountant, case history No. 30072.

First visit to our clinic was on May 10, 1985. Had a car accident 9 years previous resulting in compressive fracture of the eleventh thoracic vertebra complicated by incomplete paralysis of both lower extremities. A decompressive operation was performed just after trauma; the sensation of both lower extremities was partially recovered after the operation, and she could walk with the help of two crutches, and could gradually control bowel movement and urination. The patient received acupuncture therapy and massage for one year, and began to walk with one crutch. When exposed to cold, or in a fit of depression, old illness recurred. Examination showed no muscle atrophy in the lower extremities, but the muscular tone was increased, and there was deep hyperreflexia. Ankle clonus, and Babinski's sign positive. Mild disturbance in skin sensory function.

After 32 treatments with acupressure therapy, the tone of both lower limbs was increased. She could walk for 500 metres on one crutch, with less strain and more quickly than before. Pathological reflex: positive.

## E. Injury of Lumbar Spinal Cord

Injury of lumbar spinal cord produces paralysis of both lower limbs with sensory disturbance below the groin.

Upper section injury (L1-2): flexion of both hip joints, paralysis of femoral adductors. Atrophy of iliopsoas, sartorius, pictineus and femoral adductor muscles. The knee, ankle and toes are in a state of spasmodic paralysis. Lumbar nerve root 1.2, pains located at the groin, lateral side of gluteal part, perineum and medial aspect of the thigh. Decrease in sensory function of upper thigh above and below the groin. Hyperreflex of knee jerk, loss of cremasteric reflex. Pyramidal tract sign of lower limb positive.

Lower section injury (L3-5, S1-2): marked restraint of movements of the ankle joint, root pain at the anterior-lateral aspects of the thigh and lateral side of leg with segmental sensory disturbance of both lower limbs. Reflexes of cremasteric and biceps femoris are normal. Knee jerk and reflexes of semitendinous muscle, semimembranous muscle, gluteal reflex and ankle reflex all negative. Fecal and urinary incontinence or retention symptoms are present.

*Case report*

Liu, a male patient of 27, case No. 29164.

Fell from the third storey when working, the gluteal portion striking the ground. The 1st, 2nd, and 3rd lumbar vertebrae revealed comminuted fracture, with incomplete paralysis of both lower limbs for over 4 years. After lumbar laminectomy for decompression at the Fuyang Municipal Hospital, Anhui Province, and early osteopathic therapy, he walked on crutches. By 1984, the patient was transferred to our institute for acupressure therapy. His chief complaint on his first visit was strenuous and unstable walking with crutches, and muscle atrophy, and he was apt to tumble. Physical examination revealed drop-feet, inversion of left foot, with 3-4 grade muscle tone in both lower limbs. Dull reflex of knee-jerk and Achilles' jerk. Pathological reflex negative, slight decrease in skin sensation. After 50 sessions of acupressure treatment, muscle tone of both lower limbs increased to 4-5 degrees. He walked more steadily and the crutches were superseded by a cane. Partial recovery of atrophic muscles. Drop-foot, not completely checked.

## F. Injuries of Conus Medullaris and Cauda Equina

Injury of conus (Sacral 3, 4, 5): No obvious motor disturbance in lower limbs. Saddle shaped sensory disturbance around the anus and perineal regions, with disturbance of sexual function. Urinary and fecal incontinence or retention. Loss of bladder tone resulting in dilatation. Reflexes of the knee, ankle, sole and anus, all negative.

Injury of cauda equina: Manifestations similar to injury of lumbar spinal cord, but with flaccid paralysis. Marked atrophy of leg muscles. All reflexes below the knee negative. Sensory disturbance of nerve root distribution in the legs.

*Case report*

Case 1: Zhen, a female of 55, case No. A-838.

She was hospitalized from March 26, 1984 to May 18, 1985. Chief complaint: numbness in the left lower limb, swelling, pain and walking with difficulty for 8 years. She began feeling pain with functional disturbance in the left lower limb from 1975 onward and had received two surgical operations at neurosurgery departments in two hospitals in 1980 and 1981 respectively. A neurofibroma in the vertebral canal of the lumbo-sacral region was excised. After the operation, signs of injury to cauda equina appeared, including pain in the left lower limb, numbness and dull sensation; movement of left ankle joint was constrained. Limping when the left sole flexed at 110, with dragging steps. Difficulty in walking, with halted steps. Hyporeflexia of left knee. Achilles' jerk. Babinski's sign negative. Diagonosis: injury of cauda equina nerves (sequelae of excision of tumors in the lumbo-sacral vetebral canal).

Treatment: Acupressure therapy. The points used were Yaoyan (EX-B 7), Guan-yuanshu (BL 26), Huantiao (GB 30), Yinmen (BL 37), Weizhong (BL 40), Chengshan (BL 57), Genjian, Jiexi (ST 41), Taichong (LR 3), Zhulinqi (GB 41). The stimulation-lines Nos. 3, 4, 5, 6, and 7 of the lower extremities were selected for treatment, supplemented with passive movements of the left ankle and knee joints. After 70 sessions of treatment, the left lower limb was more stable when walking, with practically no pain. Partial recovery of sensory function of left foot. The left ankle joint could flex at an angle of 90. Swelling was gone in the left leg and foot.

Case 2: Huang, a boy of 5, admission No. 13320.

Complained of functional disturbance and soft lower extremities after operation on protrusion of sacral spinal membrane. He could not extend his knees straight or stand with his feet close together. Both feet were equino-varus. His heels could not touch the ground when walking. He walked with a swaying gesture and was incapable of running or jumping. Diagnosis: injury of the cauda equina.

After 10 sessions of acupressure therapy, both lower extremities became more powerful and the swaying walking gesture was partially corrected. He could walk and stand with both knees straight. After 50 sessions of treatment, the inversed feet were corrected, with normal function of both lower extremities and normal walking posture restored. He could jump, run, walk up and down stairs and climb a hill.

## G. Sequelae of Encephalitis

*Cause*: In the broad sense, encephalitis includes encephalitis and encephalopathy, the former refers to infection of the brain, while the latter, to encephalitis-like symptoms and pathological changes without infection. The causes of encephalitis vary. Here we only refer to sequelae of B-encephalitis, bacterial encephalitis and other infections complicated by encephalitis. According to traditional Chinese medicine, encephalitis is believed to result from evil invasion by summer dampness.

The routes of invasion are:

1. Through blood circulation;

2. Invasive and diffusive route, direct invasion of neighbouring infection from outside the cranium or through the nerve root;

3. Infection through direct or indirect contamination by instruments or foreign bodies.

*Symptoms*: Sequelae of encephalitis refers to those complicated neuropsychological manifestations which are present even 1/2-1 year after the onset of disease. The signs include disturbance in consciousness such as semiconsciousness, signs of meningeal excitation, positive tests of flexion of hip and extension of knee, and positive pathological reflexes, hemiplegia, facial paralysis, tremor and other unconscious movements. In addition: hypopsia, hypoacusis, aphasia, spasm of extremities, walking with knock-knees, loss of tendon reflex. Few cases reveal hyperreflexia of deep reflex and loss of superficial reflex. For severe cases, spasm of extremities may also occur, as well as opisthotonus or ataxia, local or general epileptic seizure.

Diagnosis: Easily made on the basis of history, signs and symptoms. Attention must be paid to the presence of complications such as epilepsis.

*Treatment*: Principle types are: encephalo-tonification, resurrection, anti-epilepsis, relaxation of tendon spasm, and activation of meridian circulation.

*Methods*

1. Acupressure with points located in the head and neck regions, trunk and extremities. For selection of stimulation lines, refer to the acupressure method for "sequelae of cerebral birth injury."

2. Anti-spasmodic and orthopedic method: refer to method for "sequelae of cerebral birth injury." Those with epilepsis are contraindicated in acupressure therapy, but, in some cases, when given antiepileptic drugs, the patient can find relief from acupressure and orthopedic therapy, by means of which epilepsis can be brought under control. However, the patient needs a longer period of treatment antiepileptic remedies.

## H. Polyneuritis

*Cause*: The commonest causes are infection and intoxication, including common cold, parotitis, diphtheria, leprosy, typhoid fever, organic compounds such as lead, arsenic carbon disulphide, alcohol, sulphonamides, faracillin and isoniagide. Other causes are metabolic disturbance and malnutrition. In traditional Chinese medicine, polyneuritis may be categorized under "Wei syndrome" which is closely related with the lung and spleen pathologically, e.g. invasion of evil-wind and heat into the lung, causing consumption of body fluid; or invasion of evil-dampness into the spleen, affecting the extremities and obstructing the meridians. All these would result in malnutrition of muscles, with "Weil syndrome ensuing."

*Symptoms*: Being a kind of bilateral, symmetrical flaccid paralysis and sensory disturbance, polyneuritis or peripheral neuritis features severe supering at the distal end of the extremities, spreading gradually upward. The insidious onset of the disease is characterized by numbness at the four extremities with prickly pain or formication, resulting in decrease or total loss of sensation over a glove or stocking-shaped area.

Disturbance of motor function reveals unstable grasping movement of the hand, decrease of muscular tone in the extremities, muscle atrophy or even flabby paralysis, drop-wrist or foot, cold, smooth, thin and dry skin, and either profuse sweating or none. As the lesion affects the respiratory muscles, there will be dyspnea in different degrees.

Tendon reflex, exaggerated in early stage and then decreased or lost totally.

*Treatment*:

Principles: Activation of *qi* and blood circulation, dredging of the meridians.

Method: Acupressure therapy.

1. Points for upper extremities: Root of nails, finger joints, Jihui, Binao (LI 14), Naohui (SJ 13), Zhima, etc.

2. Points for lower extremities: Root of the nails, toe joints, Taichong (LR 3), Zhulinqi (GB 41), Jiexi (ST 41), Lougu (SP 7), Yangjiao (GB 35), Chengshan (BL 57), Weizhong (BL 40), Qimen (LR 14), Fengshi (GB 31), Huantiao (GB 30), etc.

3. Points for the trunk: Yaoyan (EX-B 7), Guanyuanshu (BL 26), etc.

4. Points for the head and neck: Tianzhu (BL 10), Fengchi (GB 20), and pression the stimulation-lines for the upper extremity: Nos. 2, 3, 5 and 6; for the lower extremity, Nos. 1, 2, 4, 5 and 7. (Figs. 55 & 56)

The effects of acupressure on this ailment are more satisfactory in the early stages and for younger patients than they are for those with a longer course of disease and for elderly patients. For severe dyspnea, emergency aid is required; no acupressure treatment should be given.

## I. Sequelae of Infantile Paralysis

This is a sequela of poliomyelitis in children. It is unlikely to occur in adult patients.

*Cause*: It is caused by the poliomyelitis virus. After the acute stage, the paralytic extremity remains flaccid, which is characterized under "Wei syndrome" in traditional Chinese medicine, the theory of which claims it to be caused by evil wind, dampness and heat invading the lung and stomach meridians.

*Symptoms*: In its acute stage, fever and digestive and respiratory symptoms are manifested which can easily be misdiagnosed as common cold. After the fever has gone, there are irregular, asymmetrical flaccid paralyses of the extremities, mostly the lower ones, which manifest soft, paralytic, slender and cold limbs, with deformity. No sensory disturbance is present. The extent of paralysis, which varies from individual to individual, corresponds to the area of nerve innervation. The tendon reflexes exaggerate initially, decreasing and disappearing at a later stage. Deformities of the lower extremities include drop foot, talipes calcaneus, talipes valgus, talipes varus, heel foot, claw foot, overextended knee, flexing contracture of knee and hip joints or flaccid hip joints, etc.

*Treatment*:

1. Acupressure therapy: For acute and convalescent cases, gently pinch the distal points for a lengthy duration, increasing force gradually. For points around the paralytic region, more percussing and pressing is applied with greater force.

Careful examination of the tone of paralytic muscles is necessary. Full appraisal and examination of the limbs deformed as a result of disharmony between antagonistic muscle groups is also required.

Correction of deformity by means of acupressure and orthotherapy along the stimulation-lines and acupoints of the lower extremities.

a. Talipes varus: Press, knead, percuss and poke Sanyinjiao (SP 6), Lougu (SP 7), Yinlingquan (SP 9) and the stimulation-lines on the medial side of the leg.

b. Talipes valgus: Press, knead, percuss and poke Fenglong (ST 40), Yangjiao (GB 35), and the stimulation-lines on the lateral aspect of the leg; supplement by pressing the back of the foot to correct deformities such as claw, everted and inverted feet.

c. Drop-foot: Commonly seen as a result of paralysis of the anterior tibial and long extension digitis pedis muscles, leading to shortening of the belly of gastrocnemius and soleus muscles. Press and knead with light or medium force the paralytic muscles in the anterior and lateral aspects of the leg, and supplement with percussing and poking the root of the nails, toe phalanges, Jiexi (ST 41), Fenglong (ST 40), Yangjiao (GB 35), Zusanli (ST 36), and the stimulation-lines on the anterior and lateral aspects of the leg. For paralysis of the posterior aspect, press, knead and poke with medium or strong force Genjian, Chengshan (BL 57), Weizhong (BL 40) and the stimulation-lines on the posterior aspect of the leg, massage with three fingers to relieve the spasmodic muscles. (See Fig. 22) Correct foot deformity by pressing the knee and manipulating the foot. (See Figs. 21, 23, & 24) If necessary, the ankle joint may be cast in plaster in an over extension position. In some cases, satisfactory results are achieved in two weeks.

d. Over extension of the knee: For cases of flaccidity of the hamstring and gastrocnemius muscles, activate the stimulation-lines on the posterior aspect of the lower extremities, and press and knead Chengshan (BL 57), Weizhong (BL 40), Yinmen (BL 37), Biguan (ST 31), Futu (ST 32) and Qimen (LR 14). For cases of severe paralysis of both anterior and posterior muscles, the two sides should be treated at the same time. For those who cannot stand or walk due to over extension of the knee, correct with a support or rubber hoop.

e. Spasmodic flexion of the knee: Lightly press the anterior stimulation-lines and points on the thigh and press the posterior muscles of the thigh and leg with the patient in a prone position. In case the knee joint is deformed in a flexed position due to adhesion of the soft tissue, it should be released by passive extension of the joint, accompanied by manipulation. Use an external fixture with plaster cast or plaster support when necessary.

f. Contracture of hip-joint: Press the gluteal part with the patient in a prone position. Press the stimulation-lines on the lateral, anterior and medial aspects of the thigh.

g. Relaxation of hip-joint: Manipulate the stimulation-lines in the gluteal and thigh regions, the Huantiao (GB 30) point and gluteal muscles.

2. Other auxiliary treatments

The patients are encouraged to do functional exercises such as climbing, sitting, standing with support, walking, walking with crutches or sticks, jumping, squatting-and-rising, tiptoeing up and down, etc. Their relatives should knock the affected limbs moderately by hand. For the upper limb, knock mainly at the shoulder and lateral side of the elbow; for the lower limb, at the gluteal region and thigh, at the leg and around the joints. Do this 2 or 3 times daily, for 200-300 beats each time. The patients' relatives should also be taught to perform orthopedic manipulations and do these regularly.

For severe cases, when the above treatments fail due to old age or other reasons, orthotherapy with muscle-teno transfer and three-joints fusion may be necessary.

## J. Injury of Brachial Plexus

The brachial plexus is formed by the 5th, 6th, 7th, 8th cervical and the first thoracic nerves. Sometimes the 4th cervical, and second thoracic nerves also contribute to its formation. These nerves govern all the motor and sensory functions of the upper extremities with the following exceptions:

1. Motor-function: The trapezius is innervated by the 11th cranial nerve (accessory nerve);

2. Sensory function: The skin of the upper part of the deltoid muscle is innervated by the supraclavicular nerve from the cervical plexus, while a small part of the lateral skin of the arm is innervated by the intercostal brachial nerve from the third intercostal nerves.

*Causes of injury:*

Mostly caused by drawing or wrenching rather than by cutting or piercing. In case of difficult labour, the midwife's forceful separation of the foetal head and shoulder might injure the upper part of brachial plexus, causing birth paralysis. In adult patients, it may be caused by a heavy blow on the shoulder or a fall with the shoulder hitting the ground. At the time of injury, when the arm is in an abducted position, the lower part of the plexus would be affected. In case the arm is abducted and extended backward with the head deviated to the opposite side, the whole plexus would be injured. However, it is rare when only the upper or lower part is injured; usually, a mixed type of injury is found.

*Symptoms*

Typical symptoms in upper part injury (C5-6) are flaccidity of upper limb, adduction and interval rotation of shoulder joint, extension of elbow joint, supination of forearm, paralysis of infraspinatus, teres minor, deltoid, subscapular and teres major muscles, and partial paralysis of pectoris major and latissimus dorsi muscles. The brachial biceps, brachial and brachio-radial muscles are also paralyzed.

Manifestations of lower part injury of the brachial plexus (C8, T1) are paralysis of the intrinsic muscles of the hand and the digital flexion and wrist flexion muscles. In case the preganglionic fibers are affected, Horner's syndrome will occur with constriction of the pupil on the affected side and sinking of the eyeball and narrowing of the palpebral fissure.

*Injury of the tract:*

1. Injury of the lateral tract leads to paralysis of humerus, brachial muscles, coracobrachial muscle, pronator teres and radial flexor muscle of the wrist.

2. In case of posterior tract injury, the subscapular muscles and teres major are paralyzed; latissimus dorsi is partially paralyzed; deltoid and teres minor are also paralyzed; the shoulder joint is unable to rotate medially and is adducted; the wrist and fingers are unable to extend.

3. Manifestations of the injury of the medio-lateral tract are similar to the symptoms of injured median and ulnar nerves except for the flexor muscles of the wrist on the radial side and the pronator teres.

*Treatment*

Injury of brachial plexus by sharp edges is rare. Should it occur, early examination and operation are necessary.

For common injury caused by traction, the muscle tone of the whole upper limb should be carefully examined and the extent and location of the injury analyzed. Early acupressure therapy is recommended. In case treatment is unsatisfactory after six months, nerve grafting is recommended. During the operation, when contraction of the innervated muscle follows electric stimulation of the proximal end of the injured nerve, neurolysis should be performed.

1. Acupressure therapy: The points are: Binfeng (SI 12), Jianjing (GB 21), Jianyu (LI 15), Zhima, Binao (LI 14), Naohui (SJ 13), Jihui, Jianshi (PC 5), Yangchi (SJ 4), Yangxi (LI 5), Interphalangeal joints, and root of nail. The stimulation-lines are Nos. 1, 2, 3, 4, 5, and 6 of the upper limbs. Perform once daily or every other day. (See Figs. 55 & 56)

2. Supportive therapy: Hang the upper limb with the elbow flexed at 90. Prevents edema and improves blood circulation of the upper limb.

3. Functional exercise: The patient or his relatives are requested to assist with active and passive exercises of the shoulder, elbow, wrist and hand joints, so as to prevent functional degeneration due to disuse.

*Case report*

Huang, 2-month-old boy, case No. 28796.

His brachial plexus was injured by drawing of the left shoulder during delivery, with manifestations of dropping of the left upper limb, which was powerless and displayed disturbance in forearm supination. The left forearm revealed muscle atrophy and drop-wrist with reasonable grasping movement. Impression: Incomplete injury of left brachial plexus.

*Treatment*

Points for left shoulder and upper limb: Jianjing (GB 21), Jianyu (LI 15), Zhima, Binao (LI 14), Jihui, Yangchi (Sj 4), Yangxi (LI 5), root of nail, and finger joints. Stimulation-lines Nos. 2, 3, 5, and 6 of the left upper limb. Apply treatment once every other day for 30 sessions. Basically, the function of the left shoulder, elbow and wrist was recovered.

## K. Injury of Radial Nerve

The radial nerve, innervating mainly the extensors of the upper limbs including the triceps of brachium, the humero-radial muscle, supinator, extensors of the hand and fingers and abductor of the thumb, is the one most susceptible to injury among the plexus nerves. The manifestations, when injured, vary according to the location of injury.

*Causes*

Fracture of upper end of humerus, dislocation or pressure by axillary crutch. During operation, the radial nerve might be injured by the humerus head which is in an abducted position. Fracture of the groove for the radial nerve at the humerus head or osteotylus may also injure this nerve. The radial nerve might be pressed when the patient's upper limb is placed under the body, as with a comatosed patient. Besides, weapon-wounds might sever the nerve directly. The nerve can also be selectively injured by lead poisoning or alcoholism.

*Symptoms*

Manifestations of radial nerve paralysis vary, depending on the location of injury.

1. Injury of the axilla will result in total paralysis, featuring total paralysis of all the extensors of the upper limb, inability to stretch the forearm and drop-wrist. The metacarpo phalangeal joints are also unable to extend and the forearm cannot supinate when extended, except when the elbow joint is flexed by the aid of brachial biceps. Since the brachio-radialis muscle is paralysed, the elbow joint cannot be flexed when the forearm is pronated. Since the wrist joint cannot be flexed, its grasping power is diminished and the thumb cannot abduct. The sensory function of the posterior aspect of the arm is disturbed.

2. Nerve injury at the middle section of the arm manifests intact extension movement of the forearm, drop wrist, inability to extend the proximal interphalangeal joints and sensory disturbance of a very small part of the thumb and the dorsal side of the first and second interphalangeal space.

3. Never injury at the proximal section of the forearm manifests disturbance in extension of the finger but no sensory disturbance in the hand.

4. Never injury at the lower section of the forearm will mainly result in motor disturbance of the thumb and index finger without sensory disturbance.

*Treatment*

1. Acupressure therapy: Stimulate along the stimulation-lines of the arm, associated with local points. For injury of the radial nerve, line Nos. 5 and 6 of the arm are chosen; the main points are Naohui (SJ 13), Quchi (LI 11), Jihui, Yangchi (SJ 4) and

Zhangjian.

2. Auxiliary treatment: Hang the injured limb in a triangular sling with the elbow joint flexed at 90 and the wrist joint extended, so that blood circulation and functional exercise will not be affected by long-time-fixation.

3. Functional exercise: The following passive movements should be performed: extension of wrist and fingers, abduction of thumb, supination of forearm, clenching the fist, extension and flexion of the elbow joint.

Total severance of the nerve trunk (neurotomesis) should be anastomosed without delay. Acupressure therapy should be started immediately after the stitches are removed.

*Case report*

Li, female farmer, age 34, case No. 16584.

Admitted for injury of the left radial nerve; received an operation in a hospital for excision of a fibroma in the left forearm. She had drop-wrist after surgery. The metacarpo-phalangeal and proximal interphalangeal joints could not extend. The thumb cannot extend backward and was abducted. Acupressure therapy was applied. Points selected are: root of nail, finger joints, Hegu (LI 4), Yangchi (SJ 4), Yangxi (LI 5), Zhangjian, Jihui, and Quchi (LI 11). Stimulation-lines were Nos. 1, 2, 5, and 6 of the upper limbs. Treatment was applied once every other day for 15 sessions. The functions of the left wrist and the hand were recovered. (See Figs. 55 & 56)

## L. Injury of Median Nerve

The muscles the median nerve innervates are: pronator teres, pronator quadratus, flexor carpiradialis, palmaris longus, flexor digitorum sublimis, the second and third flexor digitorum profundus, flexor hallucis longus, the superficial end of flexor hallucis brevis, abductor pollicis brevis, opponens pollicis, and the first, second and third digitorum lumbricales.

*Cause*

The median nerve is not apt to be injured due to its deep location. The most common causes of injury are weapon wounds, fracture of the humerus and of the radial and ulnar bones, and wrist wounds. Carpal canal syndrome results from pressure on the medial nerve in the carpal canal, caused by excessive household work such as laundering or kneading dough.

*Symptoms*

Total paralysis of the forearm will occur if the median nerve is injured. Manifestations: inability to pronate the forearm and partial inability to flex the wrist. The thumb and the middle and index fingers cannot flex, but the ring and little fingers remain flexional (flexor digitorum profundus is innervated by the ulnar nerve). There is atrophy of the thenar muscles and abduction of the thumb in an extension position, forming the so-called "ape hand." There is loss of superficial sensation of the palmar surface of 3 1/2 fingers at the radial side, and of the dorsal surface of 2 1/2 fingers at the distal end. Severe burning pain is felt when the medial nerve is partially injured.

*Treatment*

1. Acupressure therapy: The pertinent points are root of nail, finger joints, Jianshi (PC 5), Jingqu (LU 8), Shaohai (HT 3), and Zhima. The stimulation-lines are Nos. 1, 2, and 3 of the upper limbs. (See Fig. 55)

2. Auxiliary treatment: Practise the following movements: pronation of the forearm, clenching the fist, abduction of the thumb and touching the fingertips with the thumb.

In case of complete severence of the median nerve, emergency end-to-end anastomosis is required. Acupressure therapy is recommended after the stitches are removed.

## M. Injury of Ulnar Nerve

The muscles the ulnar nerve innervates are: flexor carpi ulnaris; abductor digiti minimi; opponens digiti minimi; flexor digiti minimi brevis; interossei; the third and fourth digitorum lumbricales; abductor digitorum hallucis and flexor hallucis brevis.

*Cause*

The causes include weapon wounds; fractures and dislocations of the elbow joint; contusion due to distorted extension, flexion movements in cubitus valgus; and leprosy invasion.

*Symptoms*

They include weakened movements of the hand when flexing radially, or abducting toward the ulnar side. The thumb is unable to adduct, and the fingers cannot adduct or extend. There is extreme extension of the proximal segments of the fingers with the other segments flexed, forming the claw-hand. The fourth and fifth fingers lack strength when clenching the fist; the interossei and thenar muscles atrophy. The fingers cannot make precise, steady movements. There is partial or total loss of skin sensation of the little finger at the palmar and dorsal-ulnar aspects, and of the ring finger at the ulnar aspect.

*Treatment*

1. Acupressure therapy: The selected points are root of nail, finger joints, Shaohai (HT 3) and Zhima. Stimulation-lines are Nos. 2 and 3 of the upper limbs. Use percussing and pressing techniques methods on the points and stimulation-lines.

2. Auxiliary therapy: Advise the patient to flex and extend the fingers: for example clenching the fist and picking up pieces of paper with the thumb and index finger.

Severance of the ulnar nerve trunk will necessitate emergency end-to-end anastomosis. Acupressure therapy may be applied immediately following the removal of stitches.

## N. Injury of the Sciatic Nerve

The sciatic nerve, which is the largest nerve in the body, descends in between the greater trochanter and ischial tuberosity at the posterior aspect of the femur, after passing through the greater foramen of the ischium in front of the piriformis muscle. Reaching the lower 1/3 of the thight, it bifurcates forming the tibial nerve and the peroneus communis nerve. The tibial nerve runs through the middle of the popliteal fossa and downward at the posterior aspects of the tibia and medial mallelus into the foot. The peroneus communis runs outside the opliteal fossa and downward, lateral to the neck of the fibula, and bifurcates into deep and superficial branches at the lateral malleolus.

*Cause*

The most common causes of sciatic nerve injury are inaccurate gluteal injection, accidental wounds by sharp edge and bullet penetration. Incomplete injury of the sciatic nerve may occur after operation on meningomyelocele of the sacral-lumbar spinal cord.

*Symptoms*

Injury of the sciatic nerve in the thigh will result in paralysis of muscles below the knee, leading to drop-foot, partial disturbance in the flexion of the knee and partial or complete loss of skin sensation below the knee. Injury to the tibial nerve will result in paralysis of the flexors of the metatarso-phalangeal muscles, resulting in loss of movement of the ankle joint and plantar flexion of the toes. The foot is in an abducted, dorsiflexion position due to weakness of foot adduction. The body weight falls on the heel when walking; it is impossible to tiptoe. The reflexes of the Achilles; tendon and plantar are lost, and the sensory function of a large part of the plantar, and that of the plantar surface of all the toes, and the dorsal surface of the second, third, fourth and fifth toes are lost too. When the peroneus communis nerve is injured, drop-foot will result. The patient raises his knees as he walks, as if he is afraid to let the toes touch the ground. The foot and toes are unable to flex, abduct or pronate. The skin sensation of the dorsal surface of the foot and the anterio-lateral aspect of the leg is also lost.

*Treatment*

1. Acupressure therapy: When diagnosis indicates complete or incomplete injury of the sciatic, tibial or peroneus communis nerve, early acupressure therapy is recommended.

Points: Root of toe nail, toe joints, Taichong (LR 3), Zulinqi (GB 41), Jiexi (ST 41), Genjian, Lougu (SP 7), Yangjiao (GB 35), Chengshan (BL 57), Weizhong (BL 40), Yinmen (BL 37), Huantiao (GB 30), Guanyuanshu (BL 26), and Yaoyan (EX-B 7). Stimulation-lines: below-the-knee segments of lines No. 1, 2, 3, and 4 and the entire length of lines No. 5, 6 and 7.

Manipulate the stimulation-lines with light and moderate force; repeat percussion several times at the points. Press these points 5-10 times.

2. Auxiliary therapy: Injury of the sciatic nerve in a high position as a result of imperfect gluteal injection will result in pedis equinovarus, contracture of gastrocnemius and soleus muscles. Press the dorsal aspect of the affected foot should be performed to correct eversion and arch foot. Three-finger massage may be applied to release the contraction of the two muscles. A functional splint, such as a short-plaster cast, or a steel-wire splint, may be used to fix the ankle joint in position, or the patient can simply wear orthopedic shoes for walking.

3. During the period of acupressure therapy, an exploratory operation might be necessary if Tinel syndrome remains positive, or a positive phase wave or fibrination potential are present, indicating the total loss of conductivity of the nerve. Acupressure therapy at the distal end of the limb may begin right after the

removal of stitches. The area operated on can only be manipulated three weeks after the operation. During the recovery period, pressing the wounded nerve or the proximal end of the operational suture may evoke a sensation of formication or pain in the innervated area, indicating the growth of the nerve axis toward the distal part. For example, in a case where incomplete injury of the sciatic nerve has occurred due to incorrect gluteal injection, an area of high sensitivity appears at the femoral triangle in the course of acupressure therapy. As the therapy proceeds, the area gradually shifts downward, disappearing until it reaches the tip of the toes. This is an indication of the efficacy of the therapy.

*Case report*

Zhang, female, aged 6, case No. 20907.

Complaints: Weakness and lameness of left lower limb and drop-foot. The ailment began as a result of antibiotic injection on the left back-side when treating a common cold seven months earlier, at which time she felt extreme pain in the area of the injection, followed by numbness and convulsion all the way along the sciatic nerve down to the left sole. She walked with a limp. After medical treatment for three months, her condition improved, but she still limped and wobbled. There was extensive muscle atrophy of the left lower limb, contracture of musculii gastrocnemius and soleus, resulting in pedis equinovarus, and arch foot, and a degenerative zone of sensation scattered along the sciatic innervating area. Diagnosis: incomplete injury of left sciatic nerve. After acupressure therapy for seven months, the affected skin sensation recovered and the arched foot and equinovarus were corrected. The patient no longer experienced pain and walked with a normal gait.

**Results of Zhang's Somatossensory Evoked Potential No. 124**

| Acupressure treatment | Date of examination | Site of stimulation | Site of data recorded | Latent period | Speed of conduction |
|---|---|---|---|---|---|
| Before | 1984-4-4 | left posterior tibial nerve | thoracic 12-lumbar 1 | 33.6 ms (normal: 11.8-14 ms) | 23.2 m/s |
| | | left peroneus communis nerve | ibid. | 3.4 ms (normal: 9.1-12.6) | 17.4 m/s |
| After | 1984-10-29 | left posterior tibial nerve | ibid. | 15.0 ms | 52.0 m/s |
| | | left peroneus communis nerve | ibid. | 14.2 ms | 41.5 m/s |

*Results*

Before acupressure treatment, there was a marked prolongation of the latent period of somatosensory evoked otential and a decrease in the speed of sensation conduction. The condition returned to normal after treatment.

## O. Sciatica

As a symptom, sciatica refers to pain along the area innervated by the sciatic nerve, including the gluteal region, posterior aspect of the thigh and posterior lateral aspects of the leg and lateral side of the foot.

*Cause*

Primary sciatica (ischiatitis) is mostly caused by infection of the teeth, nasal sinus and tonsils invading the nerve sheath through blood circulation, commonly accompanied by myositis and fibrinitis. Predisposing factors are cold and rheumatism.

Secondary sciatica is caused by lesions in the tissues along the sciatic nerve, such as prolapse of the lumbo-meningeal membrane of the lumbo-sacral region, tumor and tuberculosis of the spinal column, inflammation of the sacro-iliac joint, piriformis syndrome inflammation of the uterine appendages, inflammation of the hip joint, excitation as a result of gluteal injection, strain of the soft tissues at the back of thigh, etc. Such lesions produce mechanical pressure or adhesion.

*Symptoms*

Sciatica, usually occurring unilaterally, reveals an acute onset of ischiatis, manifestating pain in the lower back, stiff-waist and severe pain appearing several days afterwards along the sciatic nerve. In some cases, ephemeral pain caused by overextending the nerve occurs whilst walking or doing exercise. The pain may aggravate after several weeks and quickly intensifies. The aching, often culminating during the night, and persistent and dull at first, may develop into a burning and stinging pain. The tender areas are: the muscles beside the lumbar vertebrae, the sacral-iliac joint, the area between the iliac tuberosity and greater trochanter, the popliteal fossa, and especially the middle of the gastrocnemius. The muscles it innervates often display flaccidity, atrophy and a decrease in muscle tone. The skin in the innervated area feels extremely numb, but there are a few objective sensory disturbances. The ankle reflex may increase in the early stage, but it generally remains normal or decreases, and disappears at the chronic or severe stage. Cases of sciatica due to intervertebral disc protrusion are likely to have a history of waist or back injury, and manifest signs and symptoms other than sciatica.

*Treatment*

1. Acupressure therapy: Locate the tender point, line and area by test-pressing with the patient in a prone position. Percuss the point and along the line with light or moderate force 5-10 times. The selected acupoints are: Genjian, Fuxi (BL 38), Chengshan (BL 57), Weizhong (BL 40), Chengfu (BL 36), Huantiao (GB 30), Yaoyan (EX-B 7), Guanyuanshu (BL 26). Percussion at these points should be strong, and be repeated adequately. Then press the tender points and lines and tense muscles 50-60 times with the patient in the best possible position to relieve pain. Manipulate the roots of the toe nails, Taichong (LR 3), Jiexi (ST 41), Lougu (SP 7), and Yangjiao (GB 35) with medium force.

2. Supplementary therapies: Rational therapies pertinent to the specific causes are necessary to ameliorate the symptoms within the shortest possible time.

Orthopedic treatment is given later on for deformities. Strengthening the lumbar and lower limb muscles by exercises, such as bending the waist, rising from a squatting position, knocking the waist and affected limbs with a fist, are recommended.

## Section II

# Diseases of the Spinal Column

## A. Stiff Neck

*Cause*

This is mainly caused by an abnormal sleeping posture or slight sprain of the neck when doing exercise or manual labour. It may also be caused by wind and cold combined, deformity, or slight disarticulation of the cervical vertebrae and spasm of relevant muscles.

*Symptom*

The neck is stiff, feels painful and sore, and cannot move freely. The acromion and the internal angle of the scapular might be affected too. Movements of the upper limbs aggravate the pain. There is muscular tenderness and spasm in the affected area, and thread-like spasmodic muscle fibers can be detected by touch. This will help locate the tender points and areas.

*Treatment*

Acupressure therapy: Lightly percuss the tender points and lines 3-5 times, then press and knead the points and lines several times. Next manipulate the neck and limb in the best possible position, i.e. moving the affected neck or limb as much as is permissible.

For stiff neck due to disarticulation, manipulate by Feng's method.

For severe and chronic cases caused by combined cold and wind, thermotherapy, traditional Chinese medicinal lotion or oral administration of herbal drugs are recommended.

## B. Cervical Vertebral Syndrome

Cervical vertebral syndrome occurs mostly amongst males between the ages of 40 and 60. Dr. Chen Zhengguang diagnoses cervical vertebral syndrome as specific diseases, including: derangement of cervical vertebrae, protrusion of cervical intervertebral disc and calcification of the posterior longitudinal ligament of the cervical vertebrae, as in the case of diagnoses for stenosis of the cervical vertebral canal and cervical rib.

*Cause*

This is a syndrome resulting from pressure or stimulation of the cervical nerve caused by various factors. The vertebras C5-6 and C6-7 are most susceptible, the cause being closely related to instances of chronic strain, degenerative lesion, wounds and rheumatoid lesions of the ligaments.

*Symptom*

Clinical manifestations vary with the location of the lesion, the severity of pressure and the tissues affected. Though cervical vertebral diseases fall into different types, such as the nerve root type, spinal-cord type, vertebral artery type and sympathetic nerve type, the mixed type is the most commonly seen.

1. Symptoms of compression of the nerve-root

The incidence of this type of the disease is high among people over 40. The onset

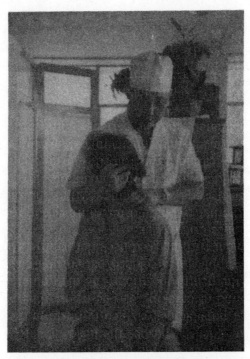

**Fig. 77  Rotational manipulation
of cervical vertebral column
introduced by Dr. Feng Tianyou**

is insidious and gradual with no previous cervical trauma. Manifestations: Persistent, recessive pain or soreness in the neck, back and shoulder (or paroxymal severe pain) when the cervical nerves are affected the pain becomes burning or stinging. The condition aggravates and the neck feels stiff and constrained when moved or with increased abdominal pressure. There is occipital pain and numbness when the upper cervical spinal nerves are excited or pressed. The upper limb of the affected side feels heavy, and powerless. Gripping strength decreases. The affected limb also feels sore, dilated and numb if pressed during sleep.

The neck might be deformed and stiffened with muscle spasm and limited mobility. There is a decrease in its physiological forward curvature, and tenderness in the post-auricle, acromion and pectoral regions, the lateral aspect of the arm, the inner-upper angle of the scapula and the region of the para-spinous process. Dragging test of the brachial plexus nerves and compressing test of the intervertebral foramen may produce positive reaction. There is radiation pain and numbness in the affected limb. When the root of cervical nerves are stimulated, a hypersensitive area may appear at the distal end. When pressure on cervical nerves is heavy and continues for a long time, the sensitivity disappears. In reflex examination, the reactions of the biceps brachi and the triceps tendon are active when the nerves are excited; the reaction drops or disappears when they are inhibited. It is recommended to record muscle strength, gripping power and muscle atrophy.

X-ray examination: Lateral position view reveals reverse, loss or diminution of physiological anterior curvature. Lesion of intervertebral disk reveals narrowing of intervertebral space, presence of spurs, mild sliding dislocation and ligament calcification. Oblique position view reveals spur of the sculus-bertebral joint pointing towards the narrowing intervertebral foramen.

X-ray findings should coincide with clinical manifestations, and diagnosis should be based mainly on the latter.

2. Symptoms of compression of the spinal cord

These are caused by pressure on the spinal cord due to protrusion of degenerative lesion of cervical intervertebral disc, spur from behind the vertebral bone, hyperplasia of small joints, hypertrophy or calcification of ligamenta flava, hypertrophic vertebral lamina or other factors causing circulatory disturbances.

*Clinical manifestations*

(a) Upper extremities: Unilateral or bilateral disturbance of motor and/or sensory function, such as soreness, swelling, numbness, burning pain, tremor and weakness affecting one, more than one, or all of the fingertips and the back or ulnar side of the hand. Similar disturbance may occur to the shoulder, scapula, upper limbs, forearm or the proximal or distal ends of the upper limbs.

(b) Lower extremities: Weakness, tremor, tendency to trip, numbness, abnormal sensations, motor or functional impairment.

(c) Homolateral symptoms: Functional disturbance, motor or sensory, in the unilateral upper or lower limbs, such as swelling, pain and muscle tremor.

(d) Alternate symptoms: Functional or motor disturbance in one upper limb and the opposite lower limb, or numbness in one upper limb and pain in the opposite lower limb.

(e) Head symptoms: Headache, dizziness or pain in the scalp.

(f) Sacral nerve symptoms: Difficult urination or defecation, abnormal sensation at glans penis, polyuria, urgent micturition, dribbling urination, weak lower limbs, backache, constipation.

*Signs*

(a) Unilateral pressure on the spinal cord:

Below the level of the lesion there is an increase in tonicity of the ipsilateral limb, with weak contraction and hyperreflex of tendons and hyporeflex of superficial reflex. Hoffmann's and Babinski's signs are positive. Clonus of patella and ankle may occur in serious cases, with contralateral sensory disturbance, the distribution of which does not always coincide with the level of lesion.

(b) Pressure on both sides of the spinal cord:

Functional disturbance, sometimes motor, is apt to occur at the early stage, whilst at the later stage, there are manifestations of varying degrees of incomplete spasmodic paralysis of the upper neuron or nerve tract, including sluggish movements and steps, unstable walking, dyspnea and confinement to bed; all limbs revealing high muscle tonicity and impaired strength, hyperreflex of tendons and hyporeflex or non-reflex to superficial stimulation. There is positive pathological reaction to sensory disturbance in varying degrees. Severe cases may reveal disturbance of sphincter muscles.

(c) Mixed type of pressure on the nerve-root and spinal-cord:

Aside from signs and symptoms of the spinal tract, there are symptoms of the cervical spinal nerve, such as numbness and pain in the shoulder, neck and upper limbs; muscle atrophy; weak reflex of biceps brachi and triceps of the arm; and weak sensation of the fingers.

(d) Mixed type of pressure on the sympathetic-spinal cord and vertebral artery:

Besides symptoms from the spinal tract, there is excitation of the sympathetic nerve and vertebral artery. (Please refer to relevant sections).

3. Symptoms of involvement of the vertebral artery

Extending from the posterior and upper aspects of the common carotid artery, the vertebral artery enters the transverse process foramen of the sixth cervical vertebra, penetrates the foramen of the transverse process of the atlas and reaches the cranium by passing through the foramen occipitalis magnum. After penetrating the duramater, it runs for a short distance, becoming the basilar artery, with bifurcations to the cerebellum, base of the pons, medulla oblongata, occipital lobe of the cerebrum, and the inner ear. The right vertebral artery might be bent when one turns one's head to the right, and consequently, the artery might become stenotic or completely blocked.

*Cause*

Effect of spur: Hyperplastic spur growth toward lateral side may stimulate the vertebral artery and cause it contract or become narrow and degenerate. Normally, the calibres of both vetebral arteries are not identical. When one of them is small and the other one is affected, spasm or obstruction is liable to occur, producing many symptoms. Lesions of the blood vessel, such as vascular sclerosis or arteritis, are apt to cause diminution of blood circulation or even obstruction.

Headache and dizziness caused by reflexive vascular spasm.

(a) Ischemia of cerebrum: When one's head turns to a certain position, dizziness, vertigo, nausea, deafness, and blurring of vision will occur. All these will disappear or greatly ameliorate when the head turns away from that position.

(b) Spinal tract symptoms: Sudden numbness of the limb, abnormal sensation, decreased gripping power, sudden tripping, or other rare symptoms, such as hoarseness, dysphasia, aphasia, paralysis of the ophthalmic muscles, ambiopia and blurred vision. Embolism of the vertebral artery may also reveal alternate limb paralysis or paralysis of all four extremities.

(c) X-ray film of cervical vertebral: Frontal radiograph shows spur at the lateral aspect of the uncus-vertebral joint of the vertebral body. The intervertebral foramen is narrow in an oblique radiograph.

4. Symptoms of sympathetic nerve involvement

There are no sympathetic nerve cells in the cervical spinal cord, nor white communicating branches in the cervical sympathetic nerve system, which depends on the gray communicating branches to communicate with the sympathetic ganglion and the white communicating branches of the 1st and 2nd thoracic sympathetic ganglion. Emanating from the sympathetic ganglion, the post ganglionic fibers spread along the anterior branch of the cervical nerve toward the pharynx, the heart, neck, head and brachial arteries. Further branches of the fibers extending to the internal carotid artery, bifurcate to the posterior part of the eye, pupil dilators, smooth muscle of the upper eyelid and inner ear.

When the cervical dura mater, posterior longitudinal ligament, intervertebral joints, cervical nerve-root or vertebral artery are affected by pressure or other injuries, reactive inflammation will reflexively stimulate the sympathetic nerve, resulting in a series of manifestations, including ptosis, blurred vision, pupil dilatation, pain in the eye-socket, headache, dizziness, pain in the occipital region and back of the neck, tachycardia, bradycardia, pericordial pain and symptoms of the peripheral vascular system including cold limbs, numbness of limbs, redness of finger-tips, fever, pain and hyperalgesia, perspirational disturbance, hypohidrosis or hyperhidrosis at the distal end of the limbs or on one side of the body. Deafness, vertigo, nystagmus, tenderness of the trigeminal nerve or greater occipital nerve, numbness of the tongue and hypoglossal disturbances may also occur.

*Treatment of cervical vertebral syndrome:*

Since the pathological changes and their manifestations are complicated and varied, the treatment should cater to both common and special symptoms to achieve satisfactory results.

(a) Acupressure therapy: Pinch the root of the nails 3-5 times. Gently press the third to sixth stimulation-lines on the affected limb and those in the back of the neck 2-3 times. Press 3-5 times each time, with light to strong pressure.

(b) Traditional Chinese orthopedic therapy:

Satisfactory results have been obtained in the last decade by applying Dr. Feng Tianyou's manipulation method for cervical vertebral syndrome. (Fig. 77)

The patient sits with the neck relaxed. The doctor supports the patient's neck with four fingers, and rests the thumb against the spinous process. He grasps the patient's mandible with the other hand, with the centre of the palm facing the chin. The doctor may also place the palmar surface of the forearm close to the mandible, holding the occipital part in his palm. Then he pushes the head upward and turns it toward the affected side to the fullest possible degree, gently pushing the spinal process forward at the same time. The sound of cracking can be heard. The patient is then requested to turn the neck back to the neutral position. The manipulation ends here.

This method is mostly applicable to elderly patients with arteriosclerosis, loosening of the intervertebral ligament with marked neck deformity. The manipulation is given once every three days or once every week.

After manipulation, the patient should restrain neck movement.

The pillow should be soft, and at the same level as the shoulder.

The manipulation should always be gentle and suited to the patient's condition. It should be steady and accurate, and never forced. During manipulation some patients might experience dizziness, vertigo and ephemeral collapse, in which case manipulation should be suspended immediately and the patient should rest. Slapping the head and back may aid recovery.

For cervical vertebral artery syndrome, the degree of neck-rotation during manipulation should be limited. In recent years, traction, localized finger massage, and manipulating the vertebra back into its original position, have all been used with satisfactory results.

For cervical vertebral syndrome of root-type, spina-cord type and sympathetic type, it is absolutely necessary to combine hand manipulation with acupressure therapy on points on the head, neck and limbs, using the same technique as that for treating paralysis.

(c) Drug therapy: Severe pain can be relieved by antipyretics and analgesics, or local-block therapy. Traditional Chinese medicine is based on the principles of activating blood, relieving stagnasis, dissipating evil wind-and-dampness, relaxing the tendons and stopping pain. Prescriptions include: Analgesic Decoction of Four items, Decoction of Radix Angelica Pubescentis and Ramnlus Loranthi, Spur Decoction and decoctions for relaxing tendons and activating the blood.

(d) Surgical operation: Surgery is performed only when non-surgical therapies have failed to eradicate severe nerve root pain or pressure syndrome. Operation is usually performed on the anterior or posterior routes and the soft tissues of the neck.

In general, there are four types of common cervical vertebral syndrome. Recently, Dr. Ni Wencai of the Institute of Orthopedics and Traumatology suggested another medullary type that singles out manifestations of injury to the medulla oblongata. The author believes that this specific type should primarily be dealt with by comprehensive therapy, supplemented by surgery only if absolutely necessary. The use of surgery should be confined to the minimum. Moreover, rotation manipulation of other cervical vertebrae should not be performed indefinitely. After 3-5 sessions, it should be substituted by massage of the neck. Acupressure therapy associated with massage as an auxiliary treatment, using techniques such as drawing the arm, pushing the neck, and other pinching, drawing and twisting techniques usually produce satisfactory results.

*Case report*

Case 1: Bai, male, 65, case No. 3343.

His first visit was on February 24, 1985. He complained of the sudden onset, four months earlier, of severe aching and limited movement of the neck, followed by numbness, pain and weakness of the right upper limb. He could not raise his right arm more than 90. He had left wrist-drop; his right hand was numb, he could not grasp things or clench his fist. There was extensive muscle atrophy in his right upper limb. Muscle atrophy was especially marked in the hand. He received hormone therapy for 10 days. The pain subsided, but other symptoms and signs remained the same.

X-ray film of the cervical vertebrae revealed hypertrophy of the anterior margin of the first, second, third, fourth, fifth, sixth, and seventh cervical vertebrae and narrowing of the intervertebral space between the sixth and seventh vetebrae. In oblique radiography, the film showed a narrowing of the fifth intervertebral foramen, osteophytosis of the posterior margin of the fifth cervical vetebra, protruding toward the intervertebral foramen. Diagnosis: Root-type of cervical vetebral syndrome.

### Results of Somatosensory Evoked Potential No. 460

| Site stimulation | Site of data recording | Results |
| --- | --- | --- |
| Right posterior tibial nerve | Lower cervical segment, ipsilateral | > 40 ms. |
| Ibid. | Midcervical segment, ipsilateral | > 40 ms. |
| Ibid. | Upper cervical segment, ipsilateral | > 40 ms. |
| Ibid. | Sensory area of foot in right cerebral cortex | > 40 ms. (normal value 33.5 + 1.5 ms.) |

After acupressure therapy for three months (36 sessions), the affected limb returned to normal. Re-examination of the somatosensory evoked potential revealed improved results as shown in the following table.

| Site of stimulation | Site of data recording | Results |
| --- | --- | --- |
| Right posterior tibial nerve | Lower cervical segment, ipsilateral | > 40 ms. |
| Ibid. | Mid-cervical segment, ipsilateral | 21.8 ms. |
| Ibid. | Upper cervical segment, ipsilateral | 27.2 ms. |
| Ibid. | Sensory area of foot in the left cerebral cortex | > 40 ms. |

Case 2: Chen, male, 39, teacher. Case No. 28865.

He complained of numbness, weakness and pain of both upper limbs, and weakness and heaviness of both lower limbs, which had lasted for over a year. He had been injured at the neck 20 years earlier, and had experienced headache immediately after the incident. He recovered without any treatment. No predisposing factor was found at the time of his admission to a hospital in Beijing, where he was hospitalized for two months. Oral hormone treatment was ineffective. Treatment in several other hospitals produced no result either. By computer tomography examination, we found that his fourth-fifth cervical vertebral suffered protrusion of the intervertebral disc, with narrowing of the spinal canal at the C-5 level.

Clinical manifestation: Mild muscle atrophy of both upper limbs, hyperreflexion of deep tendon reflex, positive pathological reflexes including Hoffmann's and Babinski's signs on both sides. No disturbance of pain sensation.

Diagnosis: Protrusion of the nucleus pulposus of C4-5 intervertebral disk and narrowing of the fifth cervical spinal canal, complicated by functional disturbance of the four limbs.

Treatment: The selected points and lines were the same as those for treating sequelae of cerebral birth injury. Manipulate the points on the head, neck, back, waist, and upper and lower limbs once every other day. Practise indefinite rotation manipulation of the cervical and limbar vertebrae once a week. After 50 sessions of treatment, soreness, pain, numbness and weakness had almost disappeared. Muscle atrophy was

## Electromyography

| Muscles | | Relaxation | | Fibrina-tion | Fascicula-tion | Mild contraction | | | Mean voltage | Heavy contraction | |
|---|---|---|---|---|---|---|---|---|---|---|---|
| | | Insert electric potential | Ortho-phase | | | Average time limit | Polyphasic wave | Changes | | Wave pattern | Peak voltage |
| Right deltoid | First visit | - | - | - | - | 12 ms. | 40% | / | 235 uv | Interference phase | 2100 uv |
| | Second visit | - | - | - | - | 10.7 ms. | / | | 344 uv | Ibid. | 2000 uv |
| Right abductor of little finger | First visit | - | + | + | - | 13.3 ms. | / | 40% | 819 uv | Mixed phase | 3000 uv |
| | Second visit | - | + | + | - | 12.4 ms. | / | | 950 uv | Interference phase | 2500 uv |

Result: Partial neurogenic injury to the right abductors of the little finger revealed amelioration in electromyograph after treatment.

partially cured. There was slight hyperreflexion of deep reflex, but pathological reflex remained unchanged. He resumed his work.

Note: It is widely known that in order to reduce pressure on the spinal canal caused by cervical vertebral stenosis, surgical operation is necessary. However, in this case, the patient improved markedly, psychologically, symptomatically and physiologically, after 50 sessions of acupressure therapy. The explanation probably lies in the improvement of blood circulation inside the spinal canal and detumescence of soft tissue, resulting in a decrease of pressure on the cervical spinal cord.

## C. Herniation of the Lumbar Intervertebral Disk

This refers to the protrusion of the intervertebral nucleus pulposus or part of the cartilage disk through a weak point in the circular ligament. When the nucleus pulposus protrudes forward or sideways into the loose part of the vertebra, forming intravertebral nodules, the protrusion does not produce any pressure on nerve tissues and is of no clinical significance. Only when the nucleus pulposus protrudes toward the vertebral canal will there be pressure on the nerve roots or the spinal marrow.

*Cause*

Two factors are responsible for the protrusion of the nucleus pulposus: degeneration of the nucleus and rupture or weakness of the circular ligament, the direct cause for this being a sudden increase in the burden on the disk or external injury to the waist. Injuries can be multiple or single. Most patients complain of a sudden attack of sprain, such as bending to carry a heavy load in an inappropriate posture, carrying a heavy load on the shoulder, bending the waist for too long, tripping, collision, contusion, etc.

*Symptoms*

Occur mostly at L5-S1, with L4-L5 next in order. The nerve roots of the lumbar segment run vertically downward, but the foramina are located at a position higher than the corresponding intervertebral spaces. Hence, the nerve roots of the same segment leave the spinal canal above the intervertebral space and the pressure is thus often on the nerve root of the next segment below.

The ailment is apt to occur in males between 20 and 40. Most cases have a history of waist pain before feeling radiating pain in one or both lower limbs. The pain usually begins from the gluteal region and extends towards the back of the thigh, posterior-lateral aspects of the leg and the back of the foot. Coughing, sneezing or over-exertion in defecation may aggravate the pain; the pain subsides or disappears after resting in bed.

In chronic cases, there is a numb area at the lateral aspect of the leg and the back of the foot. Some patients may experience difficulty in urinating or retention of urine, due to disturbance of the sphincter muscles.

*Signs*

(a) Disappearance of lumbar lordosis, revealing straight or kyphotic curvature or scoliosis toward the affected side.

(b) Spasm of para-vertebral muscles, marked limitation of bending movement, aggravated when stretching the waist, and numbness in the lower limbs.

(c) Tenderness or percussive pain of affected spinous process on one or both sides.

(d) Pain at the affected area when the carotid vein is pressed.

(e) The patient is unable to elevate the leg on the affected side more than 30; weakness in dorsal extension of the affected hallux.

(f) Atypical distribution of decreased sensory area on the affected side.

(g) Reflex:

Decrease or loss of ipsilateral knee jerk when L3-4 is affected.

Knee and ankle jerks become inconspicuous when L4-L5 is affected.

Loss of ipsilateral ankle jerk and normal knee jerk when L5-S1 is ill.

According to Dr. Jiang Weizhuang of the Institute, herniation of the lumbar intervertebral disk can be categorized into three types:

(a) Elastic type: This occurs mostly to young people with a history of sprain or other injuries. Sudden onset. Persistent clinical manifestations consist mainly of wandering pain in the waist and lower limbs. The vertebral column shows anti-pain scoliosis, with limitations of waist movement in certain directions. The scoliotic vertebral curvature may be ameliorated by resting in bed.

X-ray examination shows straightening of physiological lumbar vertebral curvature, opisthotonus, scoliosis with narrow anteriority and wide posteriority. No stenosis of intervertebral spaces or hyperosteogeny is present.

(b) Unstable degenerative type: This occurs mostly to the middle-aged. Manifestations are the same as for the elastic type. Chronic, recurrent wandering pain in the waist, mostly occurring prior to pain in the lower extremities. Sometimes, alternative, referred pain occurs in both lower extremities.

X-ray examination shows changes in the physiological curvature of the column, with loss of anterior lumbar curvature and scoliosis, narrowing of the intervertebral spaces and increased density on the edge of the vertebral end plate. The open-close movement of bending and stretching becomes wider, with slight forward or backward sliding of the vertebral body and relative looseness of that space.

(c) Proliferative stenosis type: This is the result of a long period of chronic pain in the waist and leg, such as an early waist injury. This type occurs mostly to the middle-aged and the elderly. The characteristics are: marked disturbance of nerve root perception and motor function with intermittent lameness. The changes in physiological curvature are rather fixed, and are accompanied by compensatory abnormal contour of the waist.

X-ray examination shows narrowing of the affected intervertebral space and osteophyte formation at the anterior and posterior margins of the vertebral body. The intervertebral articular process becomes hypertrophic and hyperplastic. There is asymmetrical, relative narrowing of the space between the vertebral laminae.

*Treatment*

Based on an overall analysis of signs and symptoms, Dr. Jiang proposes comprehensive treatment, including manipulation, traction, local blockage of tender points and Chinese materia medica, associated with functional exercise and surgical operation. For the past five years, out of 271 cases, 131 have received manipulation therapy, and the other 140, surgical operations.

The methods are as follows:

(a) Elastic type: The manipulations include: easing the tender point, drawing-shaking in a pronation posture, and vibrating, pushing, pressing and shaking the waist. Scoliosis toward the same side denotes that the protrusion is located at the ventral or shoulder side of the nerve-root. By traction of the pelvis in a supine position, rotate the pelvis, extend the abdomen and raise the lower extremities to facilitate the retraction of the protruding part of the disk.

(b) Unstable degenerative type: The disk loses its elasticity, just like a leaking tube. The treatment should be localized, using rotation manipulation (see Fig. 78) associated with lateral drawing and pushing to restore the vertebral body and the intervertebral joints to their normal position. The treatment relieves or removes tension of the nerve-root. By traction of the pelvis, the joint capsule, ligamenta flava and posterior longitudinal ligament are relieved and the displacement of the vertebral body is corrected. Frequent traction should be avoided to maintain the vertebral column in a relatively stable condition.

(c) Hyperplastic stenosis type: Manipulations include shaking the waist, drawing and flexing the hip joints, dividing and managing the tendons, etc.

The aim of manipulation treatment is to relax the muscles of the waist, the back and the lower limb, and relieve the adhesion and freezing of the intervertebral joints.

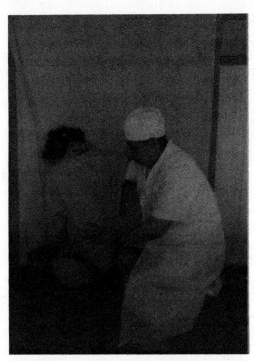

**Fig. 78   Dr. Feng Tianyou administering
rotational manipulation to lumbar portion of
spinal column with the patient in
a sitting position**

Dr. Jiang divides the affliction into three stages:

(a) Acute stage: Rest in bed, avoid strain on intervertebral disk. Manipulate from the bedside, including smoothing out the tendons, easing the points, shaking and drawing the waist and flexing the hips. To treat the tender point, apply local blocking with prednisone and procaine.

(b) Chronic persistent stage: The patient remains sitting or lying down. The manipulations mainly include rotating, supplemented by drawing, lateral pushing, and drawing-shaking in a prone (or supine) position, and other manipulations on the soft tissues. The patient is encouraged to gradually increase functional exercises and other therapeutic exercises to expedite recovery.

(c) Compensative convalescent stage: The doctor mainly gives advice for convalescence and terminates manipulation treatment. Traditional Chinese medicine aimed at generally improving health may be beneficial.

Should non-surgical treatment fail, operative exploration is recommended for an accurate diagnosis to ensure success.

## D. Derangement of Apophyseal Joints

*Cause*

Derangement of intervertebral joints, refers to displacement of intervertebral joints, incarceration of the synovial membrance and arthritis. It is common, among young people. The disease is mostly caused by acute sprain and contusion, strain or its inflammation. Out of the 3,701 cases treated in the Institute, derangement at lumbar 4 constitute 76%; at lumbar 5, 13.8%.

*Symptoms*

Manifestations include unilateral or bilateral sores and painful lumbar muscles, affecting the gluteal, thigh and sacral regions (no radiating pain), aggravated by physical exertion or change in body posture when getting out of bed.

Pain is ameliorated after starting gentle movements. Disturbance of waist function may occur in varying degrees. Tenderness of the spinous process and articular process may also occur with no radiating pain.

X-ray examination shows no positive findings. In cases of arthritis, the articular facets of the intervertebral joints become hardened, with a feathery appearance. The joint space narrows.

Diagnosis: This disease should be carefully distinguished from herniation of the intervertebral disk, piriformis injury syndrome, fracture, tuberculosis and tumor of the vertebral column.

*Treatment*

(a) Acupressure therapy: In the early stage, the affected area is severely painful with tense muscles. Gentle pressing and percussion will relieve pain and muscle spasm. Rest in bed.

(b) Orthopedic manipulation: When the acute stage is over, along with acupressure, rotate the lumbar vetebral with the patient in a sitting position to correct the displacement of the intervertebral joints and incarceration of the synovial membrane. (Please refer to relevant sections.) Acupressure therapy should be kept up to improve local blood circulation and relieve muscle spasm. (Some doctors use orthopecic manipulation as an auxiliary to acupressure therapy.)

(c) Other therapies: Local blocking of the intervertebral joint with 6-8 ml-1% procaine, plus 25 mg prednisone once weekly. In the convalescent stage, functional exercise of the back and waist muscles is recommended.

## *Section III*

# Diseases of Bones and Joints

## A. Inflammation of Soft Tissues Around the Shoulder Joint

The shoulder joint, one of the most active joints, is made up of the glenohumeral, sternoclavicular, acromio-clavicular and acromio-thoracic joints. The muscles around the joints are the deltoid, biceps, brachii triceps, brachii suprascapular, infrascapular, teres major, teres minor, scapular levator, rhomboideus, pectoralis major and pectoralis minor. The ligaments involved include the coracohumeral, glenohumeral, costoclavicular, acromioclavicular and coracoclavicular ligaments.

*Cause*

Periarthritic inflammation of the shoulder joint is caused by lesion of the joint capsule and the tissues around the joint as a result of injury, strain, degeneration, inflammation and invasion by wind, cold and dampness. It mostly occurs to females around 50 years old. In traditional Chinese medicine, it is called "fifty-year-old shoulder."

*Symptoms*

The early stage—the inflammation stage—is mainly characterized by pain, unilateral or bilateral, with local congestion and swelling, muscle spasm, tissue ischemia, degeneration and scar formation. The affliction develops into the frozen stage when the pain decreases, but the functional disturbance in the shoulder joints limits movement in all directions, including shrugging, abduction, adduction, backward stretching and rotation. In most cases, the movement is limited in only 2 or 3 directions as a result of pain or spasm of soft tissue. The longer the affliction lasts, the more extensive the invasion of tissues and the adhesion around the joint capsule, resulting in functional limitation of the multiple joints around the shoulder. Daily routines such as combing one's hair, washing one's face and dressing are all inconvenienced.

*Treatment*

Orthopedic manipulation, which moves the shoulder in four directions, in addition to acupressure therapy, has proved to be a simple and satisfactory therapy for this ailment.

*Method*

(a) With one hand the doctor holds the afflicted arm by the forearm and lifts the arm overhead anteriorly to keep the patient's shoulder in a raised position. (See Fig. 9) He then locates the tender or stiff area and applies acupressure therapy such as percussion, pressing and kneading with the other hand.

(b) Help the patient abduct the affected limb and touch the opposite auricle with the fingers. (See Fig. 11) Locate the tender area, point or soft tissue adhesion as the patient performs this movement. Press, knead or percuss the points, moving the shoulder joint at the same time.

(c) Help the patient abduct the affected shoulder to the limit, with the elbow joint flexed to 90. (See Fig. 10) Rub the forehead with the proximal portion of the forearm, the shoulder joint thus being automatically raised. Locate the tender point or soft tissue adhesion in the course of this movement and treat it with acupressure therapy. Repeat the process 7-8 times to release pain and adhesion.

(d) Help the patient stretch the afflicted arm backward to touch the spinous process with the thumb. (See Fig. 12) This movement necessitates backward stretching and pronation of the shoulder joint, flexion of the elbow joint and pronation of the forearm. While the doctor assists the patient with these movements, he locates the tender point and soft tissue adhesion and administers acupressure therapy. Repeat 5-6 times.

For acute cases, emergency treatment is necessary, such as a blocking injection. Commence combined orthopedic and acupressure therapy only after pain has been ameliorated and inflammation relieved.

*Case report*

Zhang, female, 23, case No. 32560.

Complained of pain and limited mobility in the right shoulder which had lasted for over two years. The predisposing factor was exposure to cold. Increasing pain caused insomnia and the movement of her right shoulder became increasingly limited. She also experienced weakness of the right upper limb and numbness in her right hand. She could not grasp an object tightly, thus experiencing great inconvenience in her everyday life.

Clinical examination: The right shoulder joint could only be raised to an angle of 90. Adduction, abduction, internal and external rotation of the shoulder joint were limited and caused pain. Four painful points were located around the joint. Diagnosis: inflammation of soft tissues around the right shoulder joint.

Treatment: Since the chief complaint was intolerable pain and functional disturbance, local blocking was administered by injecting 10 ml 1% procaine, plus 25 mg prednisone into the most tender point at the right insertion of deltoid and the long head of biceps brachialis. Similar injections were given to the other three tender areas. The pain was quickly relieved.

Acupressure manipulation: Jianyu (LI 15), Jianjing (GB 21), Bingfeng (LI 12), Tianzong (SI 11), and Binao (LI 14) points were selected for percussing and pressing 5-6 times. Then, the patient was helped to perform the following four movements:

(a) Raise the upper limb high in the air.

(b) Rub the forehead with her own forearm.

(c) Touch her opposite auricle via the occipital region.

(d) Rub the spinous process with her own thumb.

These movements revealed the tender points and areas and the degree of functional disturbance. Massage and acupressure treatment were given accordingly as the patient continued with the movements. The treatment was given once every three days. After six sessions, the symptoms subsided and the shoulder functions returned to normal.

## B. Rheumatoid Arthritis

A common disease of high incidence belonging to the *bi* syndrome (pain, numbness and swelling caused by wind, cold and damp, according to traditional Chinese medical theory). Seventy percent of the patients are females. It often results in disability.

*Cause*

It is a non-organic specific auto-immune disease, of which 75% of the patients reveal positive anti-IgG antibody. The latter, when combined with the patient's own IgG, forms an antigen-antibody complex, which, by adhering to the synovial membrance of the joint, activates the complement to cause inflammation.

As immunology and molecular biophysics develop, and new immunological techniques are introduced, there is increasing evidence that rheumatoid arthritis is closely related to a defect of cellular adjustment in the lymphatic system, as well as to the chronic infection of virus and mycoplasma.

Traditional Chinese medical theory maintains that the ailment is due to exogenous evil invasion and weakness in internal resistance. Evil wind, cold, dampness and heat invade the skin, muscles, joints and meridians, causing stagnation of vital energy and blood circulation which, in turn, results in pain and inflammatory reactions in the muscles and joints. Weakness in body-resistance constitutes the endogenous factor, which finds expression in loose superficial body structure and unconsolidated *Yang* vital energy. Thus, the evil exogenous factors, including evil wind, cold and dampness are apt to invade and remain in the vessels, hence the disease. The exogenous factors, as a rule, invade the body from its exterior to its interior; from the vital energy to the blood. In chronic cases, they spread through the meridians to the internal organs, including the heart, lungs, kidneys and brain.

*Manifestations:*

They may take the form of spasmodic attacks, or a continuous attack which becomes chronic. The severity varies in intensity.

Fever: In varying degrees accompanied by profuse sweating.

Arthritis: In the early stage, the affliction is intermittent, usually on one or both sides alternatively. Then it remits and worsens alternately, manifesting symmetrical pain on either side, especially during the night. The affliction may be limited to a single joint. But more often than not, it wanders to the small joints of the hands and feet, and also to the joints of the knee, ankle, hip, wrist, elbow, shoulder and vertebral column. The small joints of the four extremities often manifest deformity, osteoarthritis, limited mobility, or even bony ankylosis.

*Treatment*

No satisfactory treatment has been developed so far. Although a great deal of medical literature and research exists which deals with the ailment, and there are many medicines, both traditional and Western, which have been recommended to treat the condition, patients continue to suffer from it.

We have developed a comprehensive programme for its treatment:

(a) Oral administration of herbal drugs, supplemented by traditional Chinese orthopedic manipulation;

(b) Block therapy for the tender points;

(c) Acupressure therapy and surgical orthopedic operation.

Since any single therapy has been found ineffective, comprehensive treatment is recommended. Surgery, especially synovectomy, is not advisable unless absolutely necessary.

Acupressure therapy as a supplementary treatment:

(a) Analgesic action: Although pain in multiple rheumatoid arthritis is extensive, it is possible to locate local tender points and areas to which to apply acupressure therapy.

(b) Repellent action: The swelling at the affected joints of the wrist, hand, knee, ankle, and the dorsal aspect of the foot and hand can be treated by local percussion, pressing and light knocking. The repellent effect is very conspicuous, and in some cases, instantaneous.

(c) Relaxation of joint contraction: Fibrous adhesion in the joints of the wrist, hand, shoulder, elbow, knee, and ankle may result in limited mobility, causing malfunction. This can be effectively treated by oral administration of herbal decoction, traditional Chinese orthopedic manipulation and acupressure therapy.

(d) Prevention and treatment of muscle atrophy: Muscle atrophy, which usually occurs, may be remedied by functional exercise, associated with extensive percussion, pressing and slapping.

*Case report*

He, 75, male, a retired government employee, had suffered from rheumatoid arthritis for 2 years before treatment at the Institute. The small joints of both hands and feet and the wrist and ankle joints were all swollen, painful and seriously impaired. He could not take care of himself in daily life. Pain caused insomnia. In addition to herbal drugs, acupressure therapy was given for two months. Pain and swelling were markedly relieved. Limb functions become virtually normal. He took care of himself, slept well and had a good appetite.

## Section IV
## Congenital Diseases

### A. Congenital Torticollis

*Cause*

Mainly caused by injury at birth. A common explanation is that the foetus' sterno-cleido-mastoid muscle was excessively tracted during labour, resulting in hematoma in muscle fibers and shortening of muscles, or organized contracture of the said muscle due to hemorrhage caused by obstetrical forceps. Another explanation is that the muscle is ischemic due to an abnormal foetal position, resulting in intra-uterine ischemic spasm. Hence the disease is also known as myogenic torticollis.

*Symptoms*

The main symptom is inclination of the head and neck appearing not long after birth. One of the sterno-cleido-mastoid muscles becomes atrophic and hardened into a nucleic mass. The head can only turn sideways to a certain degree. As time goes on, the neck begins to incline toward the affected side, while the mandible turns toward the normal side and the face becomes distorted and asymmetrical. Eventually, corresponding deformity takes place in the cervical vertebrae.

X-ray examination: Antero-posterior and lateral films of cervical vertebrae should be taken to determine if there are osteopathic changes and semi-vertebral deformity.

*Treatment*

Acupressure therapy: Massage with medium force the spinous process and the stimulation-lines along both sides of the upper thoracic vertebrae; then percuss and press the stimulation-lines of the neck 2-3 times. Repeatedly massage the tense and spasmodic sterno-cleido-mastoids and press the following points: Quepen (ST 12), Yixia, Jianjing (GB 21), Tianzhu (BL 10).

For spasm of muscles in the lower face, press Bige, Yingxiang (Li 20), Sibai (ST 2), Jiachengjiang (Extra). Massage the face and push with the thumb along the courses of the facial muscles.

For mild cases, remedial therapy can be applied at home, by putting the child's head in the normal position during sleep and using a board or pillow to hold it in position, or just by hand manipulation for 3-5 minutes. Repeat 3-4 times. Persistent manipulation will yield results.

## B. Congenital Equinovarus

*Cause*

The cause of this rather common disease is still obscure. Deformities on the medial side of the affected foot, including the muscles, ligaments and bones, are all secondary degenerations.

*Symptoms*

The ailment is unilateral, sometimes bilateral, varying in severity. It more often afflicts boys, the severity increasing with age. The unilaterally affected patients walk with a limp, whilst the bilateral cases are characterized by an unsteady gait, revealing adduction of the anterior part of the foot, inversion of the whole foot, and drop-foot. The leg muscles are atrophic, with reciprocal elongation of the lateral soft tissues of the foot and ankle, and shortening of the medial ones. There is callus and synovial bursae formation on the lateral aspect and dorsum of the foot, which is in touch with the ground and carries the body weight.

*Treatment*

Apply the auxiliary therapy of acupressure. Manipulate the foot (see Figs. 23 & 24) for orthopedic treatment once every other day. When the foot is passively restored to a functional position, use a plaster-cast in boot-shape to fix it. The ankle joint should be in maximum dorsal flexion, and the foot should be in an everted, abducted position. Wear the cast for 2-4 weeks. For mild cases, fix with a plaster support or a wire-splint at night. During the day time, remove the fixture, and let the patient walk whilst holding a weight. Manipulations should not be rushed, but intensified in stages so as to avoid injuring the soft tissues.

*Case report*

Teng, 1-year-old boy suffering from left congenital equinovarus, was unable to stand up. When helped to his feet, the lateral side of his left foot touched the ground, with the heel turned upward. After 3 months of manipulation without any external fixation, he was cured. A follow-up examination after one year found him walking like a normal child.

## Section V
## Other Diseases

### A. Headache

A common symptom, with pain in the area above the eyebrows and anterior to the posterior hairline.

*Cause*

1. Diseases of the intraocranial tissues, such as encephalitis, meningitis, cerebral anoxia, intracranial tumors and concussion of the brain.

2. Diseases of the eyes, nose, ears and throat, such as paranasal sinusitis, tonsillitis, nasopharyngitis, toothache, earache, myopia, hyperopia and astigmatism.

3. Organic headache, such as migraine, nervous headache, and tonic headache.

4. Headache induced by general diseases, such as hypertension, common cold and abnormal menstruation.

5. Headache induced by cervical syndromes.

*Acupressure treatment*

Selected points: Baihui (DU 20), Fengchi (GB 20), Taichong (LR 3), Zulingqi (GB 41). For migraine, add Shuaigu (BL 8).

Method of manipulation: Percuss and press the points until the patients sweats slightly. If headache is induced by common cold, or is of the nervous type, add strong percussion of the spinal column and the stimulation-lines on either side of the spine. For frontal headache, percuss Hegu (LI 4), Taiyang (EX-HN 5,) 1), Yintang (EX-HN 3). For posterior headache, percuss Fengchi (GB 20), Tianzhu (BL 10), and press and tap the occipital region. For headache induced by cervical syndrome, turn the neck and press the points in the tender area. For general headache, press Baihui (DU 20) and knock all over the head with the fingertips.

It must be pointed out that acupressure therapy only relieves headache temporarily. The doctor must diagnose the cause and treat it accordingly.

### B. Toothache

Gingivitis, periodontitis, dento-alveolar abscess, alveolitis, cementitis, pericornitis, odontoneuralgia, pulpitis and dental caries are the causes of toothache.

According to traditional Chinese medical theory, toothache can be divided into three kinds:

1. Toothache caused by stomach fire.

Main manifestation: Severe toothache accompanied by foul breath, thirst, constipation, yellow tongue coating, forceful and rapid pulse.

2. Toothache caused by wind fire.

Main manifestations: Acute toothache with gingival swelling accompanied by chills and fever, floating and rapid pulse.

3. Toothache caused by kidney deficiency.

Main manifestations: Dull, perodic pain, loose teeth, absence of foul breath, red tongue, thready and rapid pulse.

*Acupressure Treatment*

Press Chuigen (M.A. point), Hegu (LI 4) and press and knead Zhima (M.A. point), Binao (LI 14) 3-5 times.

If pain is located in the three upper anterior teeth, press points Bige, Yingxiang (LI 20); if in the three lower anterior teeth, press Jiachengjiang (Extra), Shanglianquan (Extra); if in the five upper posterior teeth, press Xiaguan (ST 7), the upper molar eminence and the buccal region; if in the five lower posterior teeth, press Chuigen.

Press the point for 15-30 seconds, lightly at first, gradually increasing the pressure until the tender area feels numb. If the pain recurs after a few hours, repeat the treatment.

Acupressure therapy provides only temporary relief. The toothache has to be diagnosed and treated accordingly.

## C. Abdominal Pain

Abdominal pain is a symptom which is frequently encountered, often accompanied by acute or chronic diseases of the internal organs, such as stomach spasm, peptic ulcer, indigestion as a result of excessive consumption of raw and cold food, appendicitis, intussusception, acute gastroenteritis, intestinal obstruction, spasm or infarction, biliary ascariasis, etc.

*Treatment*

Acupressure manipulation can be applied for temporary relief before a diagnosis is made. Give appropriate treatment according to the diagnosis.

For epigastric pain, press points Jiuwei (RN 15), Shangwan (RN 13), Zusanli (ST 36), and the tender area on the left side of the 3-4 thoracic spinous process.

For hypogastric pain, press the points mentioned above, in addition to Geshu (BL 17), Yaoyan (EX-B 7), Qugu (RN 2), Shenque (RN 8), and Jimai (LR 12). The patient lies supine and breathes diaphragmatically. Press slowly with the thumb so as to touch the spinal cord during exhalation.

*Case report*

Patient Liu, female, 15 years old, case No. 13471.

She was taking her mother to the Institute for treatment of omalgia. Suddenly the girl felt pain in the epigastric region. She complained that such periodic attacks had occurred every week for the past five years. She was given acupressure therapy on the spot. The doctor pressed Geshu (BL 17) and the tender area on the left side of the 3-4 thoracic spinous process 5-6 times. The girl rested for about 10 minutes; the pain stopped. From then on the treatment was repeated once every three days. After 10 sessions, her periodic epigastric pain disappeared. A follow-up examination six months later showed that the recovery was complete.

## D. Hiccup

This is an involuntary spasm of the glottis and diaphragm, causing the characteristic sound. Occasional attacks of hiccups suggest a mild case which can be relieved without medication. If it persists, treatment is required. Hiccups are mostly caused by irregular diet, stagnation of the vital energy of the liver and cold in the stomach, resulting in an abnormal upward movement of the vital energy of the stomach.

*Treatment*

Press Geshu (BL 17), Zhongwan (RN 12), Neiguan (PC 6), Zusanli (ST 36), or press the tender area on the left side of the 3-4 thoracic spinous process for 30-60 seconds. This will often effectively stop the hiccups.

Supplementary points: For constipation, press Juque (RN 14); for stagnation of vital energy, press Tanzhong (RN 17) and Taichong (LR 3); for cold in the stomach, press Shangwan (RN 13). Patting the head or back 5-6 times, by surprise, may stop the hiccups right away.

## E. Nocturnal Enuresis

Nocturnal enuresis refers to involuntary discharge of the urine occurring at night or during sleep. As a morbid condition, it is mostly seen in children over the age of three, and occasionally in adults. It is mainly caused by deficiency of vital energy in the kidney, which impairs the bladder's control over urine discharge.

*Treatment*

Press the points: Shenshu (BL 23), Pangguangshu (BL 28), Zhongji (RN 3), Yaoyan (EX-B 7), Guangyuanshu (BL 26), Qugu (RN 2), Huiyin (RN 1), and Qichong (ST 30). (See Figs. 79, 80, 82, & 83).

*Manipulation procedure*

The patient lies in a supine position. Press the points: Qugu (RN 2) and Huiyin (RN 1) 4-5 times, then flex both knee joints to 90 and clap the lower abdominal region 50-60 times. (See Fig. 81) The patient then shifts to a prone position. Press points: Yaoyan (EX-B 7), Pangguangshu (BL 28) and Shenshu (BL 23) 4-5 times. Percuss along both sides of the limbar and gluteal regions. The manipulation is given once daily or once every other day. A sensation of soreness, numbness, dilation and intra-abdominal vibration should be felt at the manipulated area.

Etiologically, enuresis may also result from cerebral injuries, spinal trauma or disease, impairment of the bladder sphincter, deformity of the urinary tract, crypto-rachtis, balanitis, phimosis, urethritis, redundant prepuce, or oxyuriasis. Treatment

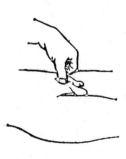

**Fig. 79    Pressing point Qugu**

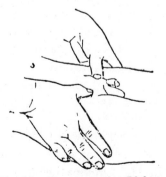

**Fig. 80    Pressing point Qichong**

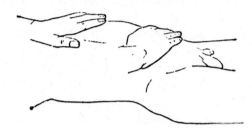

**Fig. 81   Clapping the lower abdomen**

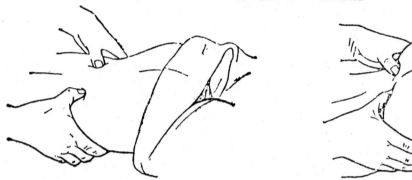

**Fig. 82    Pressing point Yaoyan**              **Fig. 83    Pressing point Guanyuanshu**

should be given accordingly.

*Case report*

Sun, male, aged 12. Chief complaint: nocturnal enuresis in the preceding 5 to 6 years. He had suffered from fractures of the tibia and fibula 6 years earlier, the treatment for which had induced frequent micturition during the daytime and bed-wetting at night. After 10 sessions of acupressure treatment, the symptoms disappeared.

## F. Common Cold

An exogenous ailment, accompanied by headache, fever, nasal obstruction, and aversion to wind as its chief manifestations. It often results from lowered superficial resistance and invasion of exogenous pathogenic factors, and may occur in any season. The manifestations can be divided into two types: wind cold and wind heat.

Wind cold manifestations: Chills, fever, anhydrosis, headache, soreness and pain of the limbs, nasal obstruction, running nose, itching of the throat, cough, hoarse voice, profuse thin sputum, thin white tongue coating, superficial and tense pulse.

*Treatment*

Press Fengchi (GB 20), Hegu (LI 4), Dazhui (GB 14). Additional points: for nasal obstruction, Yingxiang (LI 20); for headache, Taiyang (EX-HN 5); for high fever, Quchi (LI 11); for sore throat, Zengyin (Extra); for general discomfort, Dazhui (GB 14).

Prophylactic measures: Press Fengchi (GB 20) and Zusanli (ST 36) to increase immunity.

Treatment of wind heat: Press Dazhui (GB 14), Quchi (LI 11), Waiguan (SJ 5), Hegu (LI 4).

Remarks: The above treatment can also be used for other viral and bacterial infections of the upper respiratory tract as well as influenza.

Patient requires drugs besides acupressure treatment.

## G. Sunstroke

Sunstroke is an acute affliction occurring in summer, manifesting high fever, irritability, nausea, sometimes followed by collapse and loss of consciousness. The onset of this disease is due mainly to prolonged exposure to the sun or to high temperature.

There are four types of sunstroke: thermospasm, thermofailure, thermoplegia and heliosis.

*Mild case*

Headache, dizziness, profuse sweating, hot skin, heavy respiration, dire thirst, and superficial, large and rapid pulse.

*Treatment*

Press Dazhui (GB 14), Neiguan (PC 6), Quchi (LI 11), Weizhong (BL 40).

*Severe case*

Headache, dire thirst, and shortness of breath at first, followed by collapse, loss of consciousness, sweating, and deep and limp pulse.

*Treatment*

Press Baihui (DU 20), Dazhui (GB 14), Neiguan (PC 6), Weizhong (BL 40). Transfer the patient to a shady, cool and well-ventilated place. Give him intravenous infusion of 2000-3000 ml 5% glucose in normal saline, and a full dose of vitamin C daily.

According to traditional Chinese medicine, sunstroke reveals two kinds of symptom complexes.

1. Excessive symptom-complex, characterized by high fever, facial redness, shortness of breath, dire thirst, convulsion, ischidrosis, loss of consciousness, rapid pulse.

2. Insufficiency symptom-complex characterized by sweating, dizziness, weakness, cold limbs, loss of consciousness, convulsion, forceless pulse.

## H. Drowning and Its Sequelae

Drowning is a special kind of asphyxiation caused by a large amount of water entering the lung tissue and obstructing the respiratory passage, or by laryngeal spasm as a result of cold water stimulation.

However, death is not caused by asphyxiation. When a large amount of fresh water infiltrates into the blood stream, the blood is diluted and the blood volume increases. When sea water gets into the blood stream, it shifts into the pulmonary alveoli, resulting in a decrease in blood volume and a disturbance of the electrolytes. Anoxia and changes in blood volume and electrolytes will stop heart beat and respiration, followed by encephalic edema, acidosis and renal failure. Thus, administration of first-aid in cases of drowning is a complicated process.

*Clinical manifestations*

The severity of the case is closely related to the time element. A shortly drowned person will reveal cyanosis of the limbs and lips, congestive conjunctivae and spasm of the limbs. A person drowned for a longer period will reveal a cyanotic face, watery rale, respiratory noise, mouth bubbles and lung infection.

*Emergency treatment*

1. On the spot first-aid

(a) Empty the gastric content, such as water, mud, grass etc. the person is rescued from the water. Draw out the tongue and loosen the clothes. When emptying the stomach and respiratory passage, do not stop or delay cardiac massage and artificial respiration.

(b) Cardiac massage and artificial respiration. Let the patient lie in a prone position and press his or her back. A cushion or pillow should be placed under the abdomen to facilitate the outflow of water which has accumulated in the lungs and stomach. Cardiac massage on the chest wall and mouth-to-mouth artificial respiration should be performed simultaneously.

(c) Acupressure therapy. Strong stimulations should be applied to Bige, Yongquan (KI 1), Neiguan (PC 6), and Guanyuan (RN 4), to resuscitate the person.

(d) Drugs: Respiratory stimulants such as caffeine or nikethamide should be injected, in addition to administering cardiac massage. If heart-beat can no longer be heard, an intra-cardiac injection of 0.5 mg. adrenaline or 0.5-1 mg. isoprenalin should be administered.

2. Further treatment:

(a) Oxygen inhalation.

(b) Treatment of cardiac failure.

(c) Treatment of pulmonary edema and encephaledema.

(d) Correction of electrolyte disturbance and acidosis.

(e) Protection of renal function and treatment of renal failure with routine remedies.

(f) Blood transfusion for those drowned in sea-water, suffering from blood concentration and a decrease in blood volume.

(g) Antibiotics for prevention of infections.

(h) Nasal feeding for unconscious patients and use of ATP, co-enzyme A and cytochrome to improve the metabolusm of the nerve cells.

3. Treatment of sequelae of drowning. Emergency treatment of drowned persons may save their lives, but there could be a series of sequelae caused by anoxia of the brain, such as aphasia, opisthotonus, soft neck or neck spasm, hypertonus of limb muscles leading to deformities or disability or limited mobility of the limbs, profuse salivation and enuresis.

Treatments for "sequelae of cerebral birth injury" are also applicable to such cases.

## I. Shock

A syndrome of general anoxia in the tissues owing to acute circulatory failure.

Shock is characterized by apathy, restlessness, cold sweat, tachycardia, feeble pulse and dropping of blood pressure. Common causes include massive hemorrhage, severe dehydration, toxicity due to infection, wounds, anaphylactic and cardiac shock.

*Treatment*

1. Emergency treatment: Early confirmation of cause is necessary through study of the case history and physical examination, especially of the heart, the lungs and blood pressure. Apply oxygen inhalation transfusion to maintain body temperature. Apply hypothemal measures to control high fever.

Acupressure therapy: The points are Bige, (M.A. point), Zusanli (ST 36), Neiguan (PC 6), and Yongquan (KI 1). Press each point 4-5 times. Repeat after 10 minutes if necessary. The aim is to recover from collapse and regain consciousness.

2. Further treatment following emergency measures.

(a) For shock due to infection: To restore blood volume to normal and correct acidosis, a vasodiator is recommended, such as isoprenaline, dopamine, scopolamine, phenoxybenzamine and atropine. For vasoconstriction, isoprenaline and aramine are commonly used. Antibiotics should also be administered. For the prevention of renal failure manifestating oliguria and anuria, 250 ml 20% mannitol, or 25% sorbitol, should be injected intravenously.

(b) Treatment for hypovolumic shock consists mainly of emergency restoration of blood volume by injection of 500-1000 ml dextran or by blood transfusion. For massive hemorrhagic shock, blood transfusion and hemostasis are crucial; for dehydration shock, fluid should be supplied appropriately, depending upon the category to which it belongs, either the hypotonic, isotonic or hypertonic type.

(c) Allergic shock: This requires instant hypodermic injection of 1 ml of 1:1000 adrenaline, 5-10 mg of dexamethasone or 100 mg of hydrocortisone by intravenous injection, and 25 mg of phenergan by intramuscular injection. For patients with low blood pressure, intramuscularly inject or intravenously drip aramin im. or iv. or horadrenaline iv.

(d) Cardiac shock: The most common cause is acute cardiac infarction. For patients with severe angina, inject 10 mg morphine hydrochloride hypodermically, or 50-100 mg pethidine-Hcl I.M. Fluid transfusion should be dripped slowly and in small dosages, about 1/2-2/3 of the regular dosage. Digitalis is required for cardiac failure.

## J. Dizziness

Mild cases can be relieved by closing the eyes; serious ones create an illusion of body movement, like riding, sailing a boat, or traveling in a car, sometimes accompanied by nausea, vomiting and sweating.

Hypertension, anemia, neurasthenia, cerebral arteriosclerosis, diseases of the brain and inner ear, and cervical vertebral syndrome can all result in dizziness.

Traditional Chinese medicine classifies dizziness within four categories.

1. Heperactivity of the liver *Yang*.

Manifestations: Dizziness aggravated by anger, irritability, flushed face, red eyes, tinnitus, bitter taste in the mouth, red tongue with yellow coating, rapid pulse.

Acupressure treatment: Press Fengchi (GB 20), Ganshu (BL 17), Taixi (KI 3),

Xingjian (LR 2), to pacify the liver *Yang*.

2. Deficiency of vital energy and blood type.

Manifestations: Dizziness accompanied by pallor and lacklustre complexion, weakness, palpitation, insomnia, pale lips and nails, lassitude, pale tongue, thready and weak pulse. Dizziness occurs mostly after a serious disease or loss of blood and is aggravated by overwork. Loss of consciousness occurs in severe cases.

Acupressure treatment: Mildly press 5-6 times, Baihui (DU 20), Zusanli (ST 36), Guanyuan (RN 4), Sanyinjiao (SP 6), Qihai (RN 6).

3. Interior retention of phlegm dampness type.

Manifestations: Dizziness with a heavy feeling in the head and a suffocating sensation in the chest, nausea, profuse sputum, anorexia, somnolence, white sticky tongue coating, soft rolling pulse.

Acupressure treatment: Press with medium force Zhongwan (RN 12), Neiguan (PC 6), Pishu (BL 20), Baihui (DU 20), Yintang (EX-HN 3). The treatment regulates vital energy, relaxes the chest and pacifies the stomach to check vomiting.

4. Deficiency of kidney essence type.

Manifestations: Dizziness, tiredness, amnesia, soreness and weakness in waist and knees, seminal emission, tinnitus, insomnia, dreamful sleep. Manifestations of deficiency of *Yang* vitality: cold limbs, pale tongue, deep thready pulse. Deficiency of *Yin* (vital essence) is indicated by irritability, red tongue, superficial thready pulse.

Acupuncture treatment: Press, and press and knead 4-5 times Yongquan (KI 1), Shenshu (BL 23), Yaoyan (EX-B 7), Yifeng (SJ 17).

# Chapter Three
## Scientific Research on Acupressure Therapy

### Section I
### Clinical and Experimental Research on the Effect of Acupressure Therapy in Treating Sequelae of Cerebral Trauma, Cerebral Birth Injury and Incomplete Injury of the Cervical Segment of the Spinal Cord

Acupressure as a unique therapy is effective not only against common diseases but also against complex cases that baffle most orthopedists and neurologists.

A number of patients under acupressure therapy were taken at random as objects of clinical and laboratory studies at the Institute. A report follows.

### A. Clinical Data

In the last three years, 300 cases with sequelae of cerebral trauma, cerebral birth injury and incomplete injury of the cervical spinal cord were studied. Of these, 224 were outpatients; 76, inpatients.

1. Gender

**Table 1**

|  |  | Male | Female | Total |
|---|---|---|---|---|
| Sequelae of cerebral injury | Birth injury | 165 | 88 | 253 |
|  | Brain trauma | 18 | 12 | 30 |
| Sequelae of cervical spinal cord injury |  | 13 | 4 | 17 |
| Total |  | 196 (65%) | 104 (35%) | 300 |

2. Age distribution

Table 2 (see p. 116) reveals that 207, i.e. the majority of patients suffering from cerebral birth injury were between one and seven years old.

3. Causes of the injuries (see pp. 116, 117)

## Table 2

| Age | 1 | 1.1-2 | 2.1-3 | 3.1-4 | 4.1-5 | 5.1-6 | 6.1-7 | 7.1-10 | 11-15 | 16-20 | 30-40 | 41-50 | Total |
|---|---|---|---|---|---|---|---|---|---|---|---|---|---|
| Sequelae of cerebral injury   Birth injury | 11 | 47 | 52 | 24 | 34 | 24 | 15 | 18 | 21 | 6 | 1 | | 253 |
| Brain trauma | | 2 | 1 | 1 | 2 | 1 | 1 | 1 | 4 | 2 | 14 | 1 | 30 |
| Sequelae of cervical spinal | | | | | 1 | | | | | | 5 | 8 | 17 |
| Total | 11 | 49 | 53 | 25 | 37 | 25 | 16 | 19 | 25 | 11 | 20 | 9 | 300 |

## Table 3    Causes of Cerebral Birth Injuries

| Cause | Prolonged labour causing anoxia | Obstetrical instruments and anoxia | Inappropriate manipulation during delivery | Dystocia, anoxia, caesarean section | Torsion of umbical cord around neck | Breech presentation | Abruptio placentae | Total |
|---|---|---|---|---|---|---|---|---|
| Number of cases | 104 | 69 | 35 | 15 | 14 | 11 | 5 | 253 |

**Table 4    Causes of Cerebral Trauma and Injury of Cervical Spinal Cord**

| Cause | Falling | Weight squash | Traffic accident | Total |
|---|---|---|---|---|
| Number of patients | 12 | 17 | 18 | 47 |

## 4. Duration of the sequelae

The duration of cerebral birth injury was reckoned from the time of birth; and that of cerebral trauma and injury of the cervical spinal cord, from six months after the injury.

**Table 5    Duration of the Sequelae**

| Course (year) | | 0.5-1 | 1.1-2 | 2.1-3 | 3.1-4 | 4.1-5 | 5.1-6 | 6.1-7 | 7.1-8 | 8.1-10 | 10.1-20 | Total |
|---|---|---|---|---|---|---|---|---|---|---|---|---|
| Sequelae of cerebral injuries | Birth injury | 11 | 50 | 51 | 22 | 35 | 25 | 15 | 9 | 13 | 22 | 253 |
| | Brain trauma | 13 | 9 | 3 | 1 | 1 | | 1 | 1 | 1 | | 30 |
| Sequelae of cervical spinal cord injury | | 11 | 3 | 2 | | | | | | | 1 | 17 |
| Total | | 35 | 62 | 56 | 23 | 36 | 25 | 16 | 10 | 14 | 23 | 300 |

## 5. Major clinical manifestations

(a) Common clinical manifestations of injuries of the upper neuron motor system were paralysis, increased muscle tone, hyperactive tendon reflexes, diminution or loss of superficial reflexes, positive pathological reflexes and absence of muscle atrophy.

(b) Common clinical manifestations of injury of the lower neuron motor system were muscular paralysis of the injured, innervated area, decreased muscle tone, diminution or loss of tendon reflexes, muscle atrophy but no pathological reflexes.

Other clinical manifestations.

**Table 6    Functional Disturbance of Limbs**

| Affected parts | | Four extremities | Unilateral extremities | | Total |
|---|---|---|---|---|---|
| | | | Left | Right | |
| Sequelae of cerebral injury | Birth injury | 173 | 32 | 48 | 253 |
| | Brain trauma | 11 | 7 | 12 | 30 |
| Sequelae of cervical spinal cord injury | | 12 | 5 | | 17 |
| Total | | 196 (65%) | 44 (15%) | 60 (20%) | 300 |

## 6. Acupressure treatment

Prior to acupressure treatment, a comprehensive study of case histories and necessary clinical examinations was conducted. For manipulation techniques and the selection of points and stimulation-lines, please refer to Chapter II, Section I, A: Sequelae of Cerebral Birth Injury.

**Table 7    Conditions Before and After Acupressure Therapy in 240 Cases of Cerebral and Cervical Spinal Cord Injuries (patients over 2 years of age)**

| Items under observation | Sequelae of Cerebral and Cervical Spinal Cord Injuries | | | | | | |
| --- | --- | --- | --- | --- | --- | --- | --- |
| | Before treatment | Almost or completely cured | % | After treatment Condition improved | % | No change | % |
| Mental retardation | 42 | 0 | 0 | 17 | 40 | 25 | 60 |
| Dysphrasia | 62 | 0 | 0 | 30 | 48 | 32 | 52 |
| Drooling | 28 | 4 | 14 | 15 | 54 | 9 | 32 |
| Fecal and urinal incontinence | 5 | 3 | 60 | 1 | 20 | 1 | 20 |
| Opisthotonus | 10 | 2 | 20 | 7 | 70 | 1 | 10 |
| Muscle atrophy | 27 | 7 | 26 | 14 | 52 | 6 | 22 |
| Elevation of arm less than 90° | 35 | 27 | 78 | 4 | 11 | 4 | 11 |
| Difficulty in grasping | 68 | 31 | 46 | 30 | 44 | 7 | 10 |
| Inability to grasp | 64 | 31 | 48 | 22 | 34 | 11 | 18 |
| Inability to sit | 16 | 12 | 75 | 1 | 6 | 3 | 19 |
| Inability to stand | 27 | 16 | 59 | 6 | 22 | 5 | 19 |
| Inability to walk | 44 | 18 | 41 | 18 | 41 | 8 | 18 |
| Limp and sluggish gait | 111 | 49 | 44 | 44 | 40 | 18 | 16 |
| Drop foot | 89 | 46 | 52 | 25 | 28 | 18 | 20 |
| Hoffmann's sign (+) | 25 | (−) 7 | 28 | 0 | 0 | (+) 18 | 72 |
| Babinski's sign (+) | 41 | (−) 9 | 22 | 0 | 0 | (+) 32 | 78 |
| Scissor gait | 42 | 9 | 21 | 19 | 45 | 14 | 44 |

## 7. Evaluation of treatment results

Excellent: Clinical symptoms and signs basically disappeared; patient capable of complete self-care.

Good: Marked improvement, manifest spasmodic muscles relieved, patient capable of partial self-care, such as in eating, dressing and walking.

Fair: Improvement noticeable, spasmodic muscles partially relieved, recovery of disturbed functions of the limbs, patient able to take care of a small part of his/her daily routine.

Poor: Symptoms and signs showing slight improvement, slight recovery of muscle activity, muscle spasm remaining, no change in function of limbs.

Rate of effectiveness: 88%; Rate of excellent and good effect: 59%.

Amongst the 300 patients, 214 received 1-2 complete courses, 75 received 3-4 such courses, 11 received over 5 such courses.

#### Table 8   Evaluation of Acupressure Treatment Results in 300 Cases

|  |  | Excellent | Good | Fair | Poor | Total |
|---|---|---|---|---|---|---|
| Sequelae of cerebral injury | Birth injury | 60 | 85 | 75 | 33 | 253 |
|  | Trauma | 9 | 10 | 8 | 3 | 30 |
| Sequelae of cervical spinal cord injury |  | 6 | 7 | 4 |  | 17 |
| Total |  | 75 (25%) | 102 (34%) | 87 (29%) | 36 (12%) | 300 |

## 8. Results of reexamination

#### Table 9   Time of Follow-up Examination

|  |  | 3-5 months treatment | 6 months-1 year | 1.1-1.5 years | Total |
|---|---|---|---|---|---|
| Sequelae of cerebral injury | Birth injury | 16 | 54 | 18 | 88 |
|  | Trauma | 3 | 3 | 10 | 16 |
| Sequelae of cervical spinal cord injury |  | 4 |  | 9 | 13 |
| Total |  | 23 | 57 | 37 | 117 |

#### Table 10   Results upon Completion of Acupressure Treatment and Follow-up Examination

|  |  | Excellent | | Good | | Fair | | Poor | |
|---|---|---|---|---|---|---|---|---|---|
|  |  | Upon completion | Follow-up | Upon completion | Follow-up | Upon completion | Follow-up | Upon completion | Follow-up |
| Sequelae of cerebral injury | Birth injury | 40 | 46 | 26 | 29 | 15 | 7 | 7 | 6 |
|  | Trauma | 7 | 10 | 6 | 5 | 2 | 1 | 1 |  |
| Sequelae of cervical spinal cord injury |  | 4 | 6 | 6 | 4 | 3 | 3 |  |  |
| Total |  | 51 | 52 | 38 | 38 | 20 | 11 | 8 | 6 |
| Percentage |  | 44 | 53 | 32 | 32 | 17 | 9 | 7 | 6 |

There is no marked difference between the results at the end of the treatment course and those of follow-up examinations.

## B. Clinical Examination and Experimental Study

Clinical observation of the patients after acupressure treatment revealed obvious changes in the nervous, muscular and circulatory systems, as well as in the body as a whole. Laboratory studies of these changes were made.

### 1. Changes in somatosensory evoked potential (SEP)

Twenty-one adult patients and 24 5- to 10-year-old ones were examined electro-phsiologically, by computerized superposition, for their injuries in the cerebrum, cervical spinal cord and nerve root.

It was found that the latent period of (SEP) in 45 cases was prolonged, as compared with that of normal persons, with very obvious differences of statistical significance, which is helpful in determining clinical diagnosis. The 45 cases all displayed improvement after treatment; of these, 28 cases were reexamined. Results showed that the prolonged latent period was normal or nearly normal. This suggests that SEP may also serve as a quantitative index for checking therapeutic efficacy.

#### Table 11    Results of 73 Sessions of SEP Examination of 28 Cases
#### Before and After 20-100 Sessions of Acupressure Treatment

| Item examined | Time of examination | | Mean value | t value | p value |
|---|---|---|---|---|---|
| Latent period of SEP | Acupressure therapy | Before | $19.8547 \pm 5.632$ | 4.8341 | $p < 0.001$ |
| | | After | $16.0027 \pm 4.125$ | | |

SEP latent period was shortened after acupressure treatment. The difference was significant.

### 2. Study on the changes in cardiovascular functions

Twenty patients were randomly selected for examination of their cardiovascular functions, of whom 14 were suffering from sequelae of traumatic or birth wounds to the cerebrum, and the other 6 from injury to the cervical spinal cord.

*Method of examination*

Heart rate, stroke volume for each beat, peripheral resistance and blood pressure were used as indices and examined in a quiet milieu, with the patient lying supine.

Each stroke volume and peripheral resistance were estimated by measuring arterial pressure at the humeral artery; whilst the diastolic pressure was obtained at the point when the beating sound suddenly became blurred. To avoid errors, the examination was undertaken three times by the same examiner, in the same milieux, with the patient completely receptive and at ease. The mean volume was obtained by using Starr's method:

Each stroke volume = $(93 + 0.54 \times$ pulse pressure$) - (0.47 \times$ diastolic pressure $+ 0.61 \times$ age$)$

Peripheral resistance = mean pressure $\times 1332/$each stroke volume

Comparison between the value before and after a single session of acupressure manipulation showed no significant statistical difference in heart rate ($p < 0.4$), each stroke volume ($p < 0.3$) and arterial systlic pressure ($p < 0.4$). However, there was significant difference in diastolic pressure (p ‹ 0.05) and peripheral resistance (p ‹ 0.05). See Table 12 and Fig. 84.

### Table 12 Comparison of Results of Cardiovascular Functions in 20 Cases Before and After a Single Acupressure Manipulation

| Function | Measuring | Time | Mean value | t value | p value |
|---|---|---|---|---|---|
| Heart rate (beat/min) | Acupressure manipulation | Before After | 81.45 79.70 | 0.8229 | ‹ 0.4 |
| Each stroke volume (ml) | " | Before After | 60.30 64.15 | 1.8024 | ‹ 0.3 |
| Peripheral resistance (dyne sec/cm$^5$) | " | Before After | 2183.85 1948.90 | 2.2011 | ‹ 0.05 |
| Arterial systolic pressure (mmHg) | " | Before After | 108.60 112.41 | 0.82 | ‹ 0.4 |
| Arterial diastolic pressure (mmHg) | " | Before After | 76.90 70.89 | 2.1190 | ‹ 0.05 |

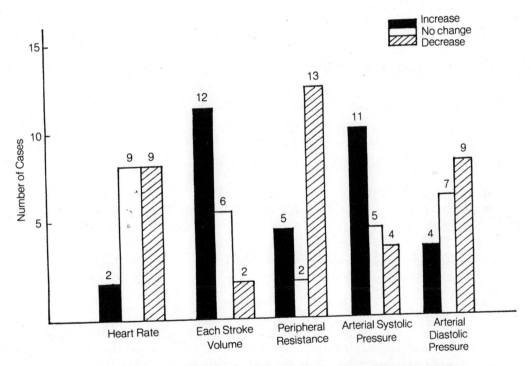

**Fig. 84 Diagram comparing results of cardiovascular function in 20 cases before and after a single acupressure manipulation**

This suggests that acupressure therapy lowers the arterial diastolic pressure, increases the pulse pressure by decreasing the peripheral resistance in the arterioles, especially in the arterial capillaries, resulting in the increase of circulatory velocity and improvement of blood circulation. (See Fig. 84)

Patients suffering from injuries to the cerebrum and cervical segment of the spinal cord, with functional disturbance of limbs, revealed a close relationship between the cardiovascular function and stagnation of vital energy and blood in the extremities. The most obvious example for this was the disturbance of peripheral blood circulation in the extremities, and evidence that the patients were apt to suffer from frostbite, cold fingers and toes, murky grey skin, dull sensation and limited mobility, indicating an increase in peripheral vascular resistance which the traditional Chinese medicine interprets as: "abnormality caused by the blocking of blood vessels, counteraction between *Yin* and *Yang*, stagnation of vital energy and blood circulation and deficiency of the meridians," which can be ameliorated by acupressure therapy.

### 3. Study on microcirculation in fingernail fold

(a) Twenty-two cases were examined for changes in fingernail fold microcirculation before and after a single acupressure manipulation. The examination was conducted with an 80-time WX-753 B microcirculation microscope produced by the Xuzhou Optical Instrument Factory. For results, see Table 13.

### Table 13

| Site examined | Change after acupressure | Person/session |
| --- | --- | --- |
| | Increase in blood circulatory velocity | 18 |
| Nailfold of fingers | Coarsening of capillary loops | 15 |
| | Increase in clarity of the capillary loop | 20 |
| | Revelation of the originally overlaid loop | 2 |
| Total | | 22 cases, 55 sessions |

The microscope had no device for recording blood circulatory velocity.

(b) Seven cases were examined by computer for changes in microcirculation in fingernail fold. Changes in circulatory velocity are indicated in the following Table 14 and Fig. 85. After acupressure manipulation, the loop calibres were found to have widened to varying degrees, the number of loops within 1 mm had increased and the degree of clarity of the loops had improved.

### 4. Study on immunology

Twenty-seven cases of 1- to 10-year-olds with sequelae of cerebral birth injury were examined for their cellular immunocompetence.

The general and local reactions after acupressure therapy, such as increase in skin temperature from 1 to 3C, reddening of the skin around the site of manipulation, general comfortable feeling, sound sleep, good appetite, more energy and greater resistance against common cold indicate that acupressure not only affects the conductivity of the nervous system, cardiovascular functions and peripheral circulation, but also improves the patient's immune function. Tests to this effect were conducted, using the double-blind method to analyse earlobe microblood (0.3-0.5 ml.) to ascertain the activated Ea-rosette and Et-rosette formation count in the T-lymphocytes.

**Table 14  Comparison of Circulatory Velocity (mm/sec.) in Capillary Loop of Fingernail Fold in 7 Cases Before and After a Single Acupressure Manipulation Lasting 20 Minutes**

| Name of Patient | Sex | Age | Acupressure manipulation Before | After | t value | p value |
|---|---|---|---|---|---|---|
| 1. Li Suqin | F | 36 | 0.240 | 0.510 | 2.975 | p < 0.05 |
| 2. Zhao Xin | M | 40 | 0.325 | 0.625 | " | " |
| 3. Dong Shufang | F | 36 | 0.241 | 0.430 | " | " |
| 4. Liu Jianlan | F | 20 | 0.300 | 0.810 | " | " |
| 5. Guo Jinlu | M | 48 | 0.730 | 0.625 | " | " |
| 6. Gao Hong | F | 18 | 0.090 | 0.220 | " | " |
| 7. Wu Jian | M | 17 | 0.229 | 0.472 | " | " |

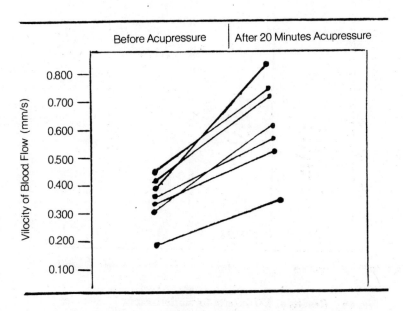

**Fig. 85  Diagram of changes in circulatory velocity in capillary loop of fingernail fold in 7 cases before and after a single acupressure treatment**

Generally, Et-rosette formation reflects the cellular immunity of the human body, whilst activated Ea-rosette formation is a subgroup in T-lymphocytes which also has an immune function and better reflects the dynamic changes in the cellular immuno-competence of the human body. (See Fig. 86)

**Table 15 Results of Rosette Formation Test in 27 Cases of 1- to 10-Year-Old Children with Sequetle of Cerebral Birth Injury**

| Rosette test | Ea | | Et | |
|---|---|---|---|---|
| | Before acupressure therapy | One month after acupressure therapy | Before acupressure therapy | One month after acupressure therapy |
| Mean value % | 29.32 | 39.07 | 58.21 | 67.71 |
| t value | | 2.1067 | | 1.9294 |
| p value | | p < 0.05 | | p < 0.05 |

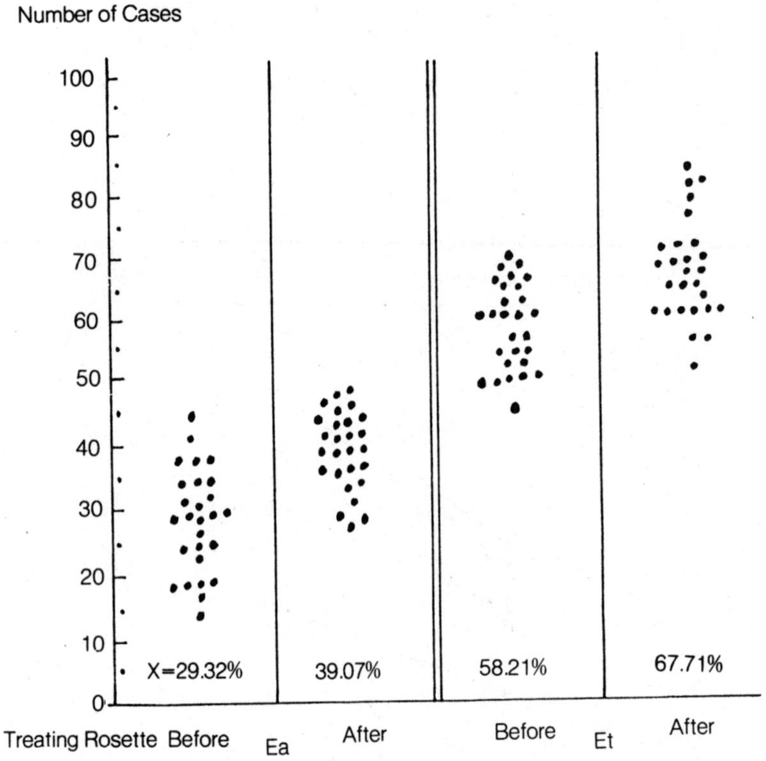

Number of Cases

**Fig. 86 Results of E-1 rosette formation test in 27 cases for sequelae of cerebral birth injury before and after five weeks acupressure treatment**

Clearly, the level of cellular immunity was elevated, especially so in the Ea count. This indicates that acupressure therapy is capable of strengthening organic resistance and expelling evil factors and is, thus, beneficial in harmonizing vital energy and blood circulation, in addition to dredging the meridians.

**Summary**

This section studies the clinical effects of acupressure therapy on three groups of patients, suffering from injury of the cerebrum; sequelae of cerebral birth injury; and sequelae of incomplete injury of the cervical spinal cord respectively.

The results of the study have shown that the clinical effect is satisfactory, the effective rate being 88%, and the rate of excellent results being 59%, of the 300 cases under study. It is widely known that cerebral paralysis is a refractory ailment. Many different therapies have been introduced, including orthopedic operations, the use of crutches or alternative supporters, orthopedic manipulation for infantile spinal deformities, acupuncture and moxibustion, massage, *tuina* manipulation, and administration of Chinese herbal medicine. All these therapies have resulted in certain improvements to the satisfaction of the patients and their families.

However, acupressure therapy, by means of manipulating the acupoints and stimulation-lines and incorporating both orthopedic manipulation and external fixation, has proved to be more effective than the other therapies mentioned above, in the treatment of cerebral and high-level partial paralysis.

The therapeutic effect was verified by measuring the somatosensory evoked potential. Examination of the cardiovascular function and microcirculation of the fingernail fold has also proved that acupressure therapy improves not only the circulation in the central nervous system, but also the microcirculation, thus providing evidence of the positive effect of acupressure therapy on the functions of the nervous and circulatory systems, whilst tests on the immune function have revealed that acupressure therapy strengthens body resistance.

These are preliminary conclusions drawn from tests on the three groups of patients under study. Future studies will focus on a selection of specific diseases to further explore the organic mechanism of acupressure therapy.

## *Section II*

## Research on the Effect of Acupressure and Its Mechanism as the Main Therapy in Treating Sequelae of Cerebral Birth Injury

In order to better probe the mechanism of the clinical effect of acupressure therapy, 300 cases of one single disease—sequelae of cerebral birth injury—were observed, of which 134 cases received follow-up examinations so as to study the long-term effect. The research focused on the therapeutic mechanism of activating blood circulation and expelling blood stagnation. Examinations were conducted on the following topics:

1. Dynamic condition of patients' cerebral blood circulation as shown by gamma-photography;

2. Microcirculation of cerebral cortex in dogs;

3. Microcirculation of patients' fingernail fold;

4. Hemorrheology in dogs.

In order to explain the substantial basis that exists for improving blood circulation by means of acupressure therapy, changes in the neurotrasmitters in blood were examined.

1. Noradrenalin (NE) in blood;

2. Adrenalin (N);

3. 5-hydroxytryptophane;

4. 5-hydroxyindale acetic acid;

5. Dopamine;

6. Activity of Cholinesterase.

The somatosensory evoked potential is a quantitative index indicating the improvement of nervous functions.

## A. Clinical Data

Of the 300 cases of sequelae of cerebral birth injuries treated in the Institute between 1983 and 1987, 280 were outpatients and 20, inpatients. Among them, 198 (66%) were male; 102 (34%) were female.

### Table 16    Age Distribution

| Age (year) | ‹ 1.9 | 2-5 | 5.1-7 | 7.1-10 | 10.1-14 | › 14 | Total |
|---|---|---|---|---|---|---|---|
| Number of cases | 38 | 174 | 45 | 28 | 7 | 10 | 300 |
| % | 12.6 | 57.4 | 15 | 10 | 2 | 3 | 100 |

### Table 17    Causes of Cerebral Birth Injuries

| Cause | Prolonged labor anoxia | Obstetrical instruments and anoxia | Inappropriate delivery manipulations | Dystocia, anoxia, ceasarean section | Torsion of umbilical cord around the neck | Breech presentation | Abruptio placenta | Total |
|---|---|---|---|---|---|---|---|---|
| Number of cases | 147 | 70 | 21 | 22 | 18 | 16 | 6 | 300 |
| % | 49 | 23.3 | 7 | 7.3 | 6 | 5.3 | 2.1 | 100 |

Ischemia and anoxia, which are the main causes of cerebral birth injuries, almost always occur simultaneously. Clinically, it is often difficult to distinguish anoxia from instrumental injuries.

The clinical manifestations of the 300 cases indicated that 50 cases (17%) had injuries in the left brain, 40 cases (13%) in the right brain, and the other 210 (70%) showed injuries on both sides.

Prior to acupressure therapy, the practitioner explained to the patient and his/her relatives the condition of the illness, the manner of manipulation, possible reactions at the beginning of the therapy, the duration of a complete course of therapy, and possible therapeutic effects, so as to ensure co-operation with the practitioner during the treatment. A complete course generally lasted 3-6 months. If the duration of treatment were to be less than that, the therapeutic effect would suffer. The manipulations varied with individual patients and their conditions.

For cerebral paralytic enuresis, we pressed Chuigen, Yingxiang (LI 20), Dicang

(ST 4), Jiachengjiang (Extra), Chengjiang (RN 24) and Lianquan (RN 23), 3-4 times. We massaged the vocal cord, hyoid bone and the small muscles above the bone 15-20 times.

For profuse salivation, we pressed Qugu (RN 2), Chongmen (SP 12), Huiyin (RN 1), Yaoyan (EX-B 7) and Guanyuanshu (BL 26), 4-5 times. We gently slapped the lower abdomen at Zhongji (RN 3), Guanyuan (RN 4), and Qihai (RN 6) points, 50-60 times. We percussed the waist and gluteal parts, and pressed Heding (EX-LE 2), whilst extending the knee joint, and Weizhong (BL 40), whilst flexing the knee joint. We pressed Yangchi (SJ 4) and Yangxi (LI 5) whilst extending the wrist and thumb, and Daling (PC 7) whilst flexing the wrist.

For patients of general weakness with extensive functional disturbances revealing few positive signs, it was enough to press the relevant points and stimulating-lines.

For sequelae of cerebral birth injuries, the following points were selected for manipulation.

Points at the head and neck regions: Baihui (DU 20), Shuaigu (GB 8), Tianzhu (BL 10), Fengchi (GB 20), Wangu (GB 12).

Points at the trunck region: Jianjing (GB 21), Geshu (BL 17), Yaoyan (EX-B 7), Guanyuanshu (BL 26).

Points in the region of the upper extremities: Zhima, Jihui, Zhangjian, Yangchi (SJ 4), Yangxi (LI 5), Hegu (LI 4), the root of the fingernail and interphalangeal joints.

Points in the region of the lower extremities: Huantiao (GB 30), Chengfu (BL 36), Yinmen (BL 37), Weizhong (BL 40), Chengshan (BL 57), Genjian, Jiexi (ST 41), Taichong (LR 3), Zulinqi (GB 41), the root of the toenail, digital joints.

Stimulation-lines: For the upper extremities, mainly lines 1, 2, 3, 5, and 6; for the lower extremities, mainly lines 1, 2, 4, 5, and 7. Manipulate these mildly and repeat the manipulation many times.

Accessory therapies:

1. Orthopedic manipulation. Deformities and functional disturbances due to cerebral birth injuries were mostly extensive and severe, and percussion and pressing the points alone could not usually bring about a complete cure. Thus, orthopedic manipulations became a necessary auxiliary. Here are some of the common orthopedic methods applied.

(a) Orthotherapy for supination disability of the forearm.

(b) Manipulations to relax the flexion contracture of the fingers.

(c) Exercise of the hip joints (frog-style) to release the spasm of the adduction muscles of the legs.

(d) Raise the stretched lower extremity and massage with three fingers to release the spasm of the posterior muscle group of the thigh.

(e) Medial and lateral rotation of the hip joint (head of femur) to remove disturbance of such movements of the thigh.

(f) Orthopedic 4-form manipulation, in a prone position, to release the spasm of the muscles of the iliac, waist regions and rectus femoris.

(g) Manipulation of the iliotibial tract, to release the spasm of the iliotibial tract.

(h) Treating drop-foot by pressing the knee.

(i) Treating drop-foot by flexing the knee at 90, pressing down on the sole and massaging with three fingers along the posterior aspect of the shank, with the patient in a prone position.

(j) Pulling the foot to treat strephexopodia and strephenopodia.

(k) Pressing the foot to treat claw-foot deformity.

Concomitant with the above 11 orthopedic operations, the spasmodic muscles were pressed and percussed at the appropriate points and along the stimulation-lines. The manipulation were performed step by step, gently and steadily in order to avoid injuring the patient.

2. External fixation

Mostly applied for treating drop-foot and talipes equinovarus. When these ailments had been checked to a certain extent by means of orthopedic and acupressure techniques and further treatment produced little or no effect, external fixation was begun by applying a long thickly-padded plaster cast to the leg for 2-3 weeks, with the knee bent at an angle of 175. The result was satisfactory. Pressure on the heel, ankle and knee was carefully avoided.

For drop-wrist, a plaster support for the forearm was used.

Steel-wire, plastic or wood splints were also used.

3. Surgical operation

The following operations were performed for functional disturbances due to sequelae of cerebral birth injuries.

(a) Lengthening of Achilles' tendon. Surgery was performed when acupressure and orthopedic manipulation lasting up to three months showed little effect. Surgery was only performed on patients over 7 years old and better still, over 10 years old. It is unsuitable for pre-school children, because the consequence of post-operative relapse could be very serious.

(b) Relaxation of femoral adductor muscles. This was to correct functional disturbance of the lower limb, owing to limitation of abduction movements of the thigh, as a result of spasm of the adductors of the femur. Surgery was performed only after 3 months of manipulation therapy had failed. Lengthening of Arhilles' tendon was performed on 7 cases, of which 3 received myotomotomy simultaneously, with satisfactory results.

Number of sessions and courses required.

Treatment was given once daily, or once every other day; 15-20 sessions made up a complete course, which was repeated 2-3 times in succession.

**Table 18    Number of Sessions Given to the 300 Cases**

| No. of sessions | 15-20 | 21-30 | 31-40 | 41-50 | 51-60 | 61-70 | 71-80 | › 80 | Total |
|---|---|---|---|---|---|---|---|---|---|
| No. of cases | 66 | 80 | 83 | 26 | 24 | 11 | 3 | 7 | 300 |
| % | 22 | 26.6 | 27.6 | 8.6 | 8 | 3.6 | 1 | 2.6 | 100 |

Most of the patients received 20-40 sessions of treatment, i.e., 2 complete courses. Experience showed that 40-60-sessions would yield better results.

**Table 19 Evaluation of Therapeutic Effect in the 300 Cases**

| Grade | Excellent | Good | Fair | Poor | Total |
|---|---|---|---|---|---|
| No. of cases | 69 | 110 | 82 | 39 | 300 |
| % | 23 | 37 | 28 | 12 | 100 |

Excellent: clinical manifestations basically disappeared; complete self-care achieved.

Good: marked amelioration of clinical manifestations; spasmodic muscles basically relieved; patient capable of partial self-care, including eating, dressing, and moving around.

Fair: Amelioration of clinical manifestations; spasmodic muscles basically relieved, partial recovery from disturbed functions of the extremities; able to take care of some daily routines such as eating, dressing and walking with assistance.

Poor: Mild improvement of symptoms and signs; slight recovery of muscle activity; spasm remained. No change in the functions of the extremities.

**Table 20 Relationship Between Effect and Patient's Condition**

| Grade | | Excellent | Good | Fair | Poor | Total | % |
|---|---|---|---|---|---|---|---|
| Severe | | 0 | 0 | 4 | 10 | 14 | 4 |
| Moderate | More serious type | 23 | 53 | 31 | 15 | 122 | 41 |
| | Less serious type | 30 | 46 | 36 | 14 | 126 | 43 |
| Mild | | 16 | 11 | 11 | 0 | 38 | 13 |
| Total | | 69 | 110 | 82 | 39 | 300 | 100 |

Severe: Serious disturbance of intellect and the functions of the extremities.

Moderate: More serious type, slight disturbance of intellect and functional disturbance of the extremities.

Less serious type: No disturbance of intellect and unilateral functional disturbance of the extremities.

Mild: No disturbance in intellect, mostly with unilateral upper or lower functional disturbance of the limb.

**Table 21    Comparative Results Before and After Acupressure Therapy in 262 Children over 2 Years Old Suffering from Cerebral Birth Injury**

| Item | Before treatment | After treatment | | | | | |
|---|---|---|---|---|---|---|---|
| | | Cure | % | Improvement | % | No change | % |
| Mental retardation | 90 | 0 | 0 | 32 | 36 | 58 | 64 |
| Dysphasia | 115 | 2 | 1 | 43 | 37 | 70 | 62 |
| Drooling | 66 | 19 | 29 | 32 | 48 | 15 | 23 |
| Weakness of neck | 50 | 4 | 8 | 25 | 50 | 21 | 42 |
| Opisthotonus | 20 | 1 | 5 | 16 | 80 | 3 | 15 |
| Muscle spasms | 71 | 5 | 7 | 54 | 76 | 12 | 17 |
| Elevation of arm less than 90 | 51 | 20 | 39 | 23 | 45 | 8 | 16 |
| Disturbance in supination of forearm | 140 | 22 | 16 | 100 | 71 | 18 | 13 |
| Drop-wrist | 63 | 7 | 11 | 39 | 62 | 17 | 27 |
| Difficulty in grasping | 138 | 35 | 25 | 88 | 64 | 15 | 11 |
| Inability to grasp | 63 | 17 | 27 | 33 | 52 | 13 | 21 |
| Inability to sit | 46 | 24 | 52 | 6 | 13 | 16 | 35 |
| Inability to stand | 65 | 36 | 55 | 8 | 12 | 21 | 33 |
| Inability to walk | 82 | 40 | 49 | 19 | 23 | 23 | 28 |
| Scissor gait | 59 | 12 | 20 | 35 | 60 | 12 | 20 |
| Drop-foot | 134 | 36 | 27 | 79 | 59 | 19 | 14 |
| Limp and sluggish gait | 194 | 47 | 24 | 124 | 64 | 23 | 12 |
| Frog type test (t) | 55 | 7 | 13 | 38 | 69 | 10 | 18 |
| Raising stretched leg limited | 41 | 16 | 39 | 21 | 51 | 4 | 10 |
| 4-form test of leg in prone position | 42 | 9 | 21 | 19 | 45 | 14 | 39 |
| Ober's sign (+) | 4 | | | 1 | 25 | 3 | 75 |
| Hyperactive biceps brachial reflex | 13 | 3 | 23 | 1 | 7 | 9 | 70 |
| Hyperactive triceps brachial reflex | 13 | 3 | 23 | 1 | 7 | 9 | 70 |
| Hyperactive styloradial reflex | 11 | 2 | 18 | | | 9 | 82 |
| Hyperactive knee jerk reflex | 22 | 3 | 14 | | | 19 | 86 |
| Hyperactive tendo achilles' reflex | 16 | 2 | 13 | | | 14 | 87 |
| Hoffmann's sign (+) | 8 | 1 | 13 | | | 7 | 87 |
| Babinski's sign (+) | 13 | 2 | 15 | | | 11 | 85 |

The results indicated in the above table demonstrated that acupressure therapy was not so effective in treating mental retardation and aphasia, but effective in curing functional disturbance of the extremities and profuse salivation. In treating tendon hyperreflexia and negative changes of pathological reflex, the result was not satisfactory only a few patients' pathological reflex turned negative.

Long-term effect of acupressure therapy

Out of the 300 cases, follow-up examination was given to 134 patients, of whom

58 were checked in the clinic and 76 returned our questionnaire.

**Table 22 Time Gap for Follow-Up Examination in 134 Cases**

| Time gap (year) | 0.5-1 | 1.1-2 | 2.1-3 | 3.1-4 | 4.1-5 | Total |
|---|---|---|---|---|---|---|
| No. of cases | 17 | 15 | 90 | 10 | 2 | 134 |
| % | 13 | 11 | 68 | 7 | 1 | 100 |

It is clear from the above results that:

1. In terms of long-term effect, the condition of the patient might take a turn for the better or for the worse, depending on post-treatment care after the patient was discharged from the hospital. Those who persisted in post-treatment exercise showed improvement, and those who didn't retrogressed.

2. The proportion of excellent and good results for long-term effect was 58% (Table 24); the corresponding figure for immediate effect was 60% (Table 19). The total effective rate was 88% in both cases.

3. It is highly disirable that the patients' family members learn manipulation skills so as to be able to carry on treatment exercises after the patient has been discharged from hospital.

Case report of sequelae of cerebral birth injuries.

Case 1. Wang Qin, male, 4 1/2 years old. Admission No. A 1604. Was admitted on September 12, 1986. Chief complaint: Functional disturbance of the right upper limb and both lower limbs for over 4 years. He was his mother's first child, born prematurely in the eighth month. Early amniorrhexis and protracted labour caused asphyxia in the uterus. After delivery, he remained cyanotic for 2 hours. His right arm was found stiff when he was 7 months old, with the right hand moving unconsciously, and still unable to hold anything at the time of admission. There was profuse salivation. He could not sit up until he was 2 1/2 years old, and had to lean against the wall when standing at the age of 3. At 3 1/2 years of age, he began to walk bowlegged, assisted by others.

Routine treatment for paralysis was given by selecting the pertinent points and stimulation-lines on the head, face, right upper limb and both lower limbs. The treatment lasted for half a year, and was administered once every two days for the first 3 months, was suspended for 3 months, and was then continued for another 3 months. Results showed relief of muscle spasm in the extremities and easier movements. The right hand could grab things. Salivation stopped. He could stand and even walk up and down stairs by himself. The effect was satisfactory. (See Figs. 87 & 88)

Case 2. Du Jing, girl, 6 years old. Admission No. A-1616.

The chief complaints were functional disturbance of right upper and lower limbs for over 6 years. Because of premature amniorrhexis, she was delivered after a two-day labour, with intra-uterine anoxia. her parents found her walking with abnormal gait. She couldn't hold things with her right hand. CT examination in several children's hospitals revealed malacia lesion at the left base of the cerebrum, with maldevelopment

## Table 23   Changes in the Grading of Therapeutic Effect in Follow-Up Examination

| Before follow-up examination | Excellent | | | | Good | | | | Fair | | | | Poor | | | | Total |
|---|---|---|---|---|---|---|---|---|---|---|---|---|---|---|---|---|---|
| Changes in grading | no change | good | fair | poor | excellent | fair | poor | no change | excellent | good | poor | no change | excellent | good | fair | no change | |
| | 19 | 14 | 8 | 2 | 11 | 10 | 4 | 22 | 2 | 9 | 3 | 18 | 0 | 2 | 3 | 7 | 134 |
| No. of cases | 43 | | | | 47 | | | | 32 | | | | 12 | | | | 134 |
| % | 32 | | | | 35 | | | | 24 | | | | 9 | | | | 100 |

## Table 24   Evaluation of Results of Follow-Up Examination

| Effect | Excellent | Good | Fair | Poor | Total |
|---|---|---|---|---|---|
| No. of cases | 32 | 47 | 39 | 16 | 134 |
| % | 23 | 35 | 30 | 12 | 100 |

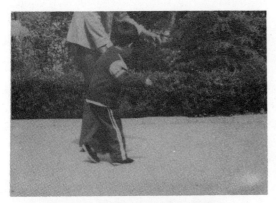

**Fig. 87    Walking with help before acupressure therapy**

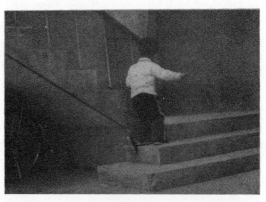

**Fig. 88    After six months of acupressure therapy, Wang Qin can walk up and down flights of stairs by himself**

of the left cerebrum. Results of acupuncture treatment for a year, were not satisfactory. Several months of treatment with encephalo-tonic failed. She was transferred to the Institute.

Pre-treatment examination: The right fingers were clumsy, with poor coordination of sophisticated finger movements. She couldn't tiptoe with her right foot, which was inverted, and swung in a circular movement when walking.

After receiving 3 months of acupressure therapy, supplemented with orthopedic manipulation of the right upper and lower limbs, and external fixation treatment for the right lower limb, both limbs recovered. (See Figs. 89 & 90)

## B. Experimental Research

**1. Observation of the changes in the somatosensory evoked potential (SEP) of patients suffering from sequelae of cerebral birth injury after treatment with acupressure therapy**

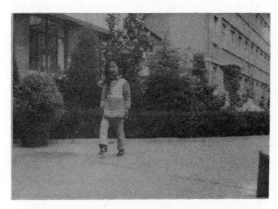

**Fig. 89    Lame in right leg before treatment**

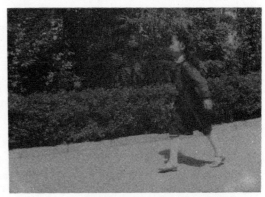

**Fig. 90    Normal gait after three months of acupressure plus orthopedic manipulation**

Sixteen cases of sequelae of cerebral birth injury, 6 female and 10 male, of age ranging from 2 to 10 years old, averaging 5, were randomly selected.

*Method of examination*

(a) After diagnosis, the first SEP examination was given before acupressure therapy. The latent period and stimulation voltage were recorded.

(b) Acupressure therapy was given according to a clinical routine. The number of sessions ranged from 20-90, averaging 55 times.

(c) The second SEP examination was given about 2 months later; the time gap varied according to the state of recovery of the functions of the extremities. The results were compared with those of the previous examination and recorded statistically.

*Process of SEP*

The patient lies supine in a state of complete relaxation, so as to avoid interference by the electromyograph. Stimulate the medial nerve at the palmo-wrist side with the bipolar electrode of a Japanese SEM-4101 stimulator, with a rectangular wave of single pulse type. The wave length was 0.2 ms and the frequency 1 Hertz, the intensity of efferent voltage was so adjusted that only the contraction of the muscles of the thenar eminence was visible. The other electrode was placed at the sensory area of the hand in the cerebral cortex, so as to receive the electric signal evoked by the stimulation. The latent period from the beginning of stimulation up until the appearance of evoked potential, and the stimulating voltage were recorded.

The acupressure routine for sequelae of cerebral birth injury was applied.

(a) Basic acupressure manipulation (pressing, percussing, pinching, tapping, etc.) supplemented by orthopedic manipulation were applied to the points on the head, neck, trunk and extremities and along the stimulation-lines. Each session usually lasted for 20 minutes, performed once daily or once every other day, for a course of 15-20 sessions.

(b) For the location of points and stimulation-lines over the whole body, see Figs. 55, 56 and 57.

After many sessions of acupressure therapy, the stimulating voltage threshold would markedly drop, which indicated the gradual recovery of the sensory function of the patient's nervous system. Increasing response to external stimulation coincided with the alleviation of clinical symptoms.

*Discussion*

(a) The latent period of SEP in patients suffering from sequelae of cerebral birth injury, before receiving acupressure therapy, was markedly longer than that in healthy persons of the same age. The latent period would shorten markedly after repeated acupressure treatment, and the stimulating voltage threshold would also drop noticeably. This demonstrated that acupressure therapy was capable of improving the conductive function of the nervous system and elevating its sensitivity to stimulation. This tallied with the recovery of sensory and motor functions of the body after acupressure treatment, and may thus serve a diagnostic purpose, in addition to providing us with a means of making quantitative evaluations concerning therapeutic efficacy.

(b) The reason why acupressure therapy improves the conductive functions of the nervous system and increases its sensitivity may be related to a comprehensive mechanism involving the activities of the enzyme system, the endocrine system, and neurotransmission—a field that is open to further investigation.

*Results*

(a) The latent period of SEP in 16 cases shortened by 2.35 ms on average, with very significant statistical differences. (See Table 25)

**Table 25    Comparative Results of SEP Examination in 16 Cases**

| Parts examined | Acupressure session | Mean value ± SD | t value | p value |
|---|---|---|---|---|
| Median nerve at the wrist to the head sensory area of the opposite cerebral cortex | Before | 18.63 ± 5.25 ms | | |
| | 20-90 times | | 3.18 | < 0.01 |
| | After | 16.28 ± 2.46 ms | | |

The conductive function of the nervous system was strengthened and the reaction to outside stimuli was stronger after treatment.

(b) The minimal stimulating voltage required to produce the contraction of the thenar muscles in the second examination was 7.65 v. lower than in the first examination. P < 0.05, showed a significant statistical difference. See Table 26.

**Table 26    Comparison of SEP Examination Minimal Stimulation Voltage**

| Item | Acupressure session | Mean value ± SD | t value | p value |
|---|---|---|---|---|
| Stimulating voltage in SEP examination | Before | 69.06 ± 17.53 v | | |
| | 20-90 times | | 2.20 | < 0.05 |
| | After | 61.41 ± 13.39 v | | |

## 2. Impact of acupressure therapy on the microcirculation of the pia mater of the cerebral cortex in dogs

Acupressure as an effective therapy for sequelae of cerebral birth injury has been found to accelerate peripheral blood circulation and improve microcirculation in the nail fold. However, its influence on microcirculation in the cerebral tissues remains unexplored. The present study investigates, by means of direct observation, its influence on the velocity of microcirculation in the pia mater of the cerebral cortex.

*Subjects and methods*

Seventeen healthy dogs, weighing 14-20 kg. each, 13 male and 4 female, were anesthetized with 3% Na-pentobarbital by intraperitoneal injection with a dosage of 40 mg/per kg. KW for craniotomy. The operated dogs lay on the lateral side with their heads slightly fixed in a horizontal position. A curved incision was made on the left side, beginning from the root of the left zygomatic process, proceeding along the posterior margin of the eyebrow arch, ascending in an arc toward the median frontal line, proceeding along the mid-occipital line posteriorly toward a point 3 cm. anterior to the greater occipital protruberance, and then curving downward to end at the upper aspect of the external auricle.

Incise the skin and subcutaneous tissues and turn the curved flap downward. Isolate and sever the temporal muscles and fascia in a downward direction along the incision. After thorough hemostasis, expose the major portions of the left temporal, parietal and frontal bones. The point for trephining was located 1.5 cm lateral to the lower left of the line linking the inner canthus and the end of the great occipital protuberance. A $2 \times 1.5$ cm$^2$ rectangular window was made after trephining and manipulated with bone scissors. Incise the dura mater upon careful hemostasis to expose the anterior and posterior sigmoidal gyri of the left frontal lobe. On the posterior gyrus a deep pial vessel of 10 u in diameter was selected for observing the velocity of blood flow and its volume.

China-made WX-753 B type microcirculation microscope and WDX-811 type capillary tachometre and apparatus for measuring vascular diameter were used.

(a) Within an hour after craniotomy but prior to acupressure, the velocity of blood flow was measured 4 times. The average figure was treated as a basic value of the velocity of cerebral capillary blood flow.

(b) Imitated acupressure treatment for human hemiplegia (unilateral hind and anterior limb, spinal column) was administered for 20 minutes.

(c) Within an hour after acupressure therapy, the velocity of blood flow in the same capillary was measured 4 times. The mean value of blood flow velocity before and after acupressure was obtained for statistical study.

After the experiment was completed, the dogs were disposed of and their brain tissue was examined to confirm the exact location of the recorded area.

*Results*

(a) Anatomical examination of the dead dogs revealed that the sites recorded and observed were all located in the middle area of the cerebral-cortical sigmoid gyri.

(b) The velocity of the blood flow in the deep pial capillaries in the recorded area was much accelerated after acupressure manipulation. In the 17 dogs, the mean value of velocity was 0.27 mm/sec. before manipulation. It rose to 0.5 mm/sec. after manipulation, an increase of 0.23 mm/sec. on average, or 185%, the P value being ‹ 0.01, a difference of statistical significance. (Figs. 91 & 92)

**Table 27    Changes in Blood Flow Velocity in the Cerebral Capillaries
of Dogs, Before and After Acupressure Treatment**

| Number of animals | Velocity before acupressure | Velocity after acupressure | t value | p value |
|---|---|---|---|---|
| 17 | 0.27 ± 0.09 mm/sec. | 0.50 ± 0.23 mm/sec. | 4.9 | ‹ 0.01 |

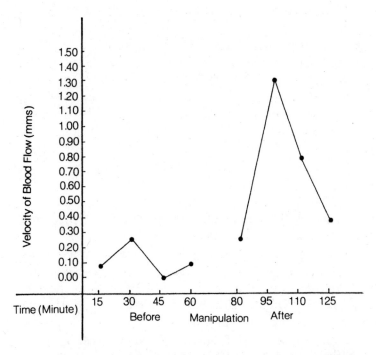

**Fig. 91    Changes of microcirculation of pial mater of cerebral cortex in 15th dog, before and after once (20 min.) acupressure manipulation**

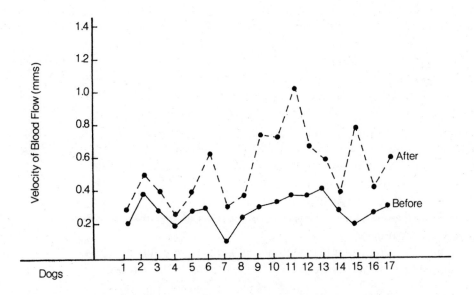

**Fig. 92    The changes of microcirculation of pial mater of cerebral cortex in 17 dogs, before and after once acupressure manipulation (20 min.)**

(c) No gender-related difference was found in the above changes.

*Discussion*

(a) The changes in the cerebral cortical pial capillaries reflect the changes inside the cortex. The cortical branch of the cerebral artery ramifies into arteriola on the surface of the pia mater and nourishes it. However, most of the arteriola penetrate the pia mater and enter the brain tissues. These arteriola nourish the brain tissues as well as the superficial white layer. That is to say, the vascular bed in the pia mater and that in the cerebral cortex share a common artery, are anatomically inseparable and have similar innervation. It is, therefore, anatomically and physiologically sound to use the pial capillary as an indicator to interpret capillary changes in the cerebral cortex as well as in the whole brain.

(b) Improvement of microcirculation in the posterior sigmoid gyrus of the cerebral cortex not only explains the recovery of motor function in patients, but also reflects the hemodynamic changes in the frontal, parietal and temporal lobes of the cerebral cortex. In terms of speciogenesis, the sigmoid cortical gyrus of dogs is isogenic and iso-functional with the central-anterior gyrus of humans. That is to say, the posterior signoid gyrus is the sensory I area in dogs. Since injury to the sensory I area of the human cerebral cortex results in the spasmodic paralysis of the opposite extremities, it is reasonable to presume that improvement of blood circulation in this area is conducive to the recovery of motor function. In view of the fact that the blood supply in the cortex of the frontal, parietal, temporal and insular lobes, comes mainly from the branches of the internal carotid system, it can be hypothesized that acupressure therapy not only improves the microcirculation of the posterior sigmoid gyrus, which is one of the frontal gyri, but also improves the circulation in other areas supplied by the internal carotid artery. It therefore stands to reason to attribute the clinical effects of acupressure therapy on movement, sensation and intellect to the improvement of blood circulation and nutrition of the area supplied by the internal carotid artery.

*Conclusion*

The experiments demonstrated that acupressure stimulation improved the microcirculation of brain tissue which, in turn, strengthened the nutritional condition and oxygen supply of the cerebral cortex as well as the whole brain, and accelerated the clearance of metabolic wastes. This eventually led to a series of metabolic changes in the brain tissue, which may possibly offer a substantial basis for strengthening functional compensation and "arousing the sleeping neurons." In other words, acupressure therapy cured sequelae of birth injury through the improvement of cerebral microcirculation. Naturally, this is by no means the only mechanism of the therapeutic effect of acupressure treatment.

**3. Research on the hemodynamics of sequelae of cerebral birth injury before and after acupressure treatment**

Acupressure treatment of sequelae of cerebral birth injury in the Institute over the years has scored a total effective rate of 88%, the proportion of excellent results being 60%.

As part of the effort to probe into the mechanism of the therapy, research on the hemodynamics in such patients has been conducted with assistance from the Central

Hospital of the Ministry of Aeronautic Industry. Results of cerebral scanning with nuclein r-scintiphotographs were studied on computer to discover the changes in cerebral hemodynamics in 15 patients suffering from sequelae of cerebral birth injury before and after acupressure therapy. It was found that after 28-60 sessions of the therapy, the patients' cerebral blood volume showed an average increase of 30%, which represented a significant statistical difference (P ‹ 0.05). This led to the postulation that the increase of blood volume and circulation in the cerebrum has a close connection with acupressure treatment. The finding was conducive to understanding the mechanism of acupressure.

The results of observation are presented below.

*Materials and methods*

(a) 15 patients suffering from sequelae of cerebral birth injury, 9 male and 6 female, were selected randomly. The patients showed motor and sensory disturbance of varying degrees. The ages of the patients ranged from 2 to 10, with an average age of 5.

(b) An imported nuclein scanner with a V77-200 type gamma ray camera was used. After an adequate dosage of nuclein Na 99 m TC 4 was injected rapidly into the cubital vein, a cerebral tachogram was obtained by taking successive orthophoric photographs of the cerebrum with an r-scinti camera. The cerebral blood volume was processed by a computer to obtain the data required.

(c) After pre-treatment examination, acupressure therapy was given. Re-examination was made after acupressure. The patients were given 20-60 sessions of acupressure therapy, averaging 39 sessions, using the basic manipulation techniques (pressing, percussing, pinching and tapping) along the stimulation-lines and at the points on the head, neck, trunk and extremities. Orthopedic manipulation (such as manipulation of the tendons of the finger, orthotherapy for supination disability of the forearm, treatment of the foot by pressing the knee and extending the hip joints) was incorporated. One session was given each day, each session lasting 20 minutes.

For the positions of points and stimulation-lines, please refer to Figs. 32-56.

*Results*

(a) After acupressure therapy, the ratio value per sec of blood volume increased by 30% in 15 cases. The statistical difference was significant. (Fig. 93)

**Table 28   Changes in Cerebral Blood Volume Before and After Acupressure Therapy in 15 Cases**

| Item examined | Acupressure therapy | | Mean value ± SD | t value | p value |
|---|---|---|---|---|---|
| Cerebral blood volume | 28-60 sessions | Before | 0.63 ± 0.24 | 2.68 | ‹ 0.05 |
| | | After | 0.93 ± 0.48 | | |

The above Table 28 and Fig. 93 demonstrate that acupressure therapy increases the cerebral blood volume and improves blood circulation.

(b) None of the 15 patients revealed any stenosis, obliteration or deformities of

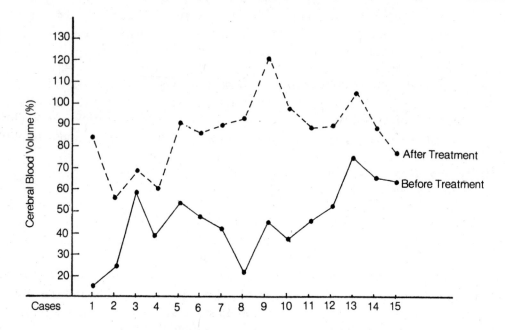

**Fig. 93    Determination of cerebral blood volume before and
after 28-60 times acupressure therapy
in 15 cases with sequelae of cerebral birth injury**

the cerebral artery except one who had stenosis of the left internal carotid artery at
the extracranial section.

This suggests that ischemia and anoxia, which are among the most common causes
of cerebral birth injury, also increase the fragility and permeability of the endothelia
of the cerebral blood vessels and cause further damage to them. However, it seems
unlikely that this would cause abnormality in the morphology of the cerebral artery.

*Discussion*

1. Being a harmless examination, the nuclein scanning of the hemodynamics of the
cerebrum doesn't cause any discomfort to the patient. Compared with other methods
such as ultrasomography, EEG, encephalo-angiography, pneumo encephalogram and
ventriculography, this scanning technique has certain advantages for the purpose of
locating intracranial lesions. Since this is an advanced technique and produces definite
quantitative results. It is used as an indicator for the presence or absence of morpho-
logical deformity of the cerebral blood vessels and for appraising the clinical efficacy
of acupressure therapy.

2. The function of the cerebrum is closely related to the supply of blood and
oxygen and the metabolism of the brain tissue. In a healthy person, the cerebrum only
takes up 2% of the total body weight, but it consumes 15% of the total cardiac blood
output, and 20% of the oxygen consumption of the whole body. Insufficient blood and
oxygen supplies might cause functional disturbances of the brain, resulting in a series
of pathological changes. Since the level of tolerance to ischemia and anoxia in
newborns is very low, and their cerebral blood flow is very rich, exceeding 100ml/

100g/M (for adults, the figure is 50ml/100g/M), most of the babies suffering from sequelae of cerebral birth injury were more or less in an ischemic and anoxic condition during delivery. Naturally, anoxia and ischemia constitute one of the main causes of multi-functional disturbances in such patients.

Study of the 15 cases indicated that the improvements in somatic and motor function, or its partial recovery, coincided with the increase of blood flow and the improvement of microcirculation in the cerebrum after acupressure therapy. This could well be one of the main mechanisms of the therapy.

3. The adjustment of cerebral blood flow is a complicated process. Under normal circumstances, there is a self-adjusting relation between the cerebral blood flow and its perfusion pressure. The cerebral blood flow can remain relatively stable even when there is a moderate change of blood perfusion pressure. In the human body, when blood perfusion pressure varies between 65-140 mmHg, the cerebral blood flow remains stable. There is also a close relation between intracranial pressure and cerebral blood perfusion pressure, the latter would fall following an increase of the former. The adjusting mechanism fails to work as soon as the intracranial pressure falls below 60 mmHg.

Changes in $CO_2$ within the body also influence cerebral blood flow through the variation of PH values of cerebrospinal or extracellular fluids. The cerebral blood flow increases as $CO_2$ increases and oxygen supply decreases, and vice versa.

Thus, blood perfusion pressure, intracranial pressure, $CO_2$ and oxygen contents are the main factors influencing cerebral blood flow. However, the specific mechanism of acupressure therapy that influences the increase of cerebral blood flow has yet to be determined.

It is highly possible that by exciting the acupoints and stimulation-lines, acupressure treatment causes changes in the release of neurotransmitters and the functional activities of the body, relaxes the soft tissues and muscles of the craniocerebral region, lowers its tension, and dilates the blood capillaries and arteriolae, thereby lowering intracranial pressure and increasing cerebral blood perfusion. Proceeding from this hypothesis, it seems plausible that further studies will be able to clarify the effect of acupressure therapy upon body functions and the release of neurotransmitters. This approach might lead to further clarification of the mechanism of acupressure therapy.

**4. Changes in microcirculation of the fingernail-fold before and after acupressure therapy in cases suffering from sequelae of cerebral birth injury**

The changes in the microcirculation of the fingernail-fold before and after one single session of acupressure therapy in 16 cases of sequelae of cerebral birth injury were studied. It was found that 20 minutes after the manipulation, the velocity of blood flow in the fingernail-fold increased by 0.128 mm/sec. which is of very significant statistical significance ($P < 0.01$), indicating that acupressure therapy might exert an influence on microcirculation in the body. A report on the results follows.

*Materials and methods*

(a) The 16 cases were selected randomly; age 4-20, average age 10; 6 were male, 10 female.

(b) The following Chinese-made instruments were used, a WDX-811 capillary hemotachometer and diametrometer, a WX-B microcirculation microscope, and a black-and-white monitor television.

(c) Before examination, the patient was told to relax for 20 minutes. Blood pressure, heart rate, pulse, body temperature and skin temperature at fingernail fold were taken under room temperature at 20 °C. Thus all physiological and pathological influences on microcirculation were excluded.

(d) Method of observation: The circulatory velocity of the left cyclomicrocirculation of the fingernail fold was measured four times at 15 minute intervals. The average value was taken. After 15 minutes, an acupressure therapy routine (see Chapter II, treatment of sequelae of cerebral birth injury) was administered for 20 minutes. The same microcirculation was measured and statistically compared with the pre-acupressure value. (See Figs. 94 & 95)

*Results*

The velocity of microcirculation in the fingernail fold in 16 patients increased after acupressure, with a mean value of 0.128 mm/sec., p ‹ 0.01, showing a very significant statistical difference.

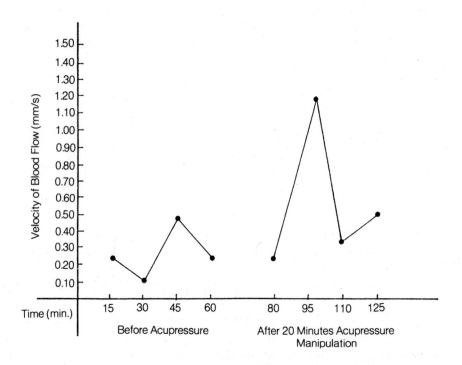

**Fig. 94    Yao, female 10 years old, examination of microcirculation of fingernail fold before and after a single acupressure manipulation**

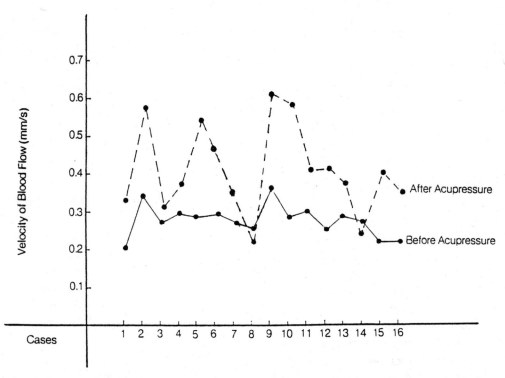

**Fig. 95    Changes in microcirculation of fingernail fold before and after a single acupressure manipulation (20 min.) in 16 cases with sequelae of cerebral birth injury**

**Table 29    Changes in the Microcirculation of the Fingernail Fold in 16 Patients Before and After Acupressure Therapy**

| Issue examined | Acupressure therapy for 20 minutes | Mean value ± SD | t value | p value |
|---|---|---|---|---|
| Microcirculation velocity of the nail-fold | Before | 0.275 ± 0.046 mm/sec. | | |
| | | | 4.65 | ‹ 0.01 |
| | After | 0.403 ± 0.116 mm/sec. | | |

The fact that the diameter of the capillaries before and after acupressure showed no significant change indicates that the therapy might have increased oxygen and blood supply by increasing the velocity of microcirculation in the body and thus improving blood circulation, and this might be one of the mechanisms of acupressure therapy.

*Discussion*

**Table 30    Changes in Microcirculation in the Fingernail Fold of 2 Groups of Patients**

| Year | 1985 | 1989 |
|---|---|---|
| Cases | Old traumatic high incomplete paraplegia | Sequelae of cerebral birth injury average age 10 years old |
| Number of patients observed | 7 adults | 16 children |
| Method of observation | Observation was made once before acupuncture and once afterwards, and the results were compared | Observation was made 4 times before acupressure and 4 times after, and the mean value was compared |
| Result | An increase of 0.27 mm/sec. after treatment, $p < 0.05$ | An increase of 0.12 mm/sec. after treatment, $p < 0.01$ |

(a) The difference between the 1985 and 1987 projects regarding the nature of the disease, the number of subjects observed and the methods of observation used, led to different results, which is of special significance to the study of the mechanism of acupressure therapy in the treatment of sequelae of cerebral birth injury.

(b) Most cases of sequelae of cerebral birth injury were accompanied by functional disturbance of the body and secondary muscular atrophy. Throughout the duration of the illness, the three symptoms generally co-existed, viz. neurotropic disturbance, disturbance in blood circulation, and disturbance as a result of disuse. They formed a vicious circle through interaction. For instance, prolonged nutritional disturbance in the endothelial cells of the blood vessels would impair their function, resulting in decreased blood supply to the affected extremity and, consequently, the exacerbation of its functional disorder.

As one of the basic physiological infrastructural phenomena and an integral part of blood circulation, microcirculation is being widely used as an indicator in the study of blood circulation in organisms. The velocity of blood flow is a major indicator of the hemodynamics of the body. Clinical experience has revealed that after acupressure therapy, the velocity of microcirculation in the fingernail-fold markedly increases, which seems to considerably improve the microcirculation in the affected limb, thereby ameliorating muscular atrophy and speeding up the recovery of the functions of the extremities. This, it appears, is one of the mechanisms of the effect of acupressure therapy.

(c) Four main factors affect the velocity of microcirculation in the fingernail-fold:
—Degree of constriction or dilation of the capillary loop.
—Level of blood pressure and cardiac output.
—Afferent and efferent resistance of the capillary loop.
—Blood viscosity.

Past experience has shown that acupressure therapy accelerates blood flow because it lowers the peripheral resistance of the arterioles, especially that of the micro-arteries, thereby increasing pulse pressure and lowering diastolic pressure in the arteries. Moreover, the therapy decreases the viscosity of plasma and whole blood in experimental dogs. It is obvious that the mechanism of the acupressure effect is closely related to the improvement in microcirculatory flow.

However, the regulation of microcirculation is a complex process involving neural and humoral adjustment and local, humoral feedback adjustment, as well as special regulation under the control of the neuro-humoral mechanism. Further exploration should be focused on the mutual relations between these complex processes.

(d) According to traditional Chinese medicine, "blood stagnation" is a symptom indicating that blood is not flowing smoothly, either generally or locally, or that there is blood existing outside its circulatory pathway, and acupressure therapy has the function of "activating blood circulation and removing stagnant blood." The TCM judgement is still another vindication of the therapy's effectiveness in accelerating microcirculatory flow and improving blood circulation.

### 5. Effect of acupressure therapy on the hemorrheology of dogs

The mechanism of acupressure therapy in treating sequelae of cerebral birth injury may have something to do with "activating blood circulation and expelling hemostagnation." In this section, attempts were made to observe acupressure's effects on dogs, with respect of changes in plasma viscosity, vicosity of whole blood, rate of thrombocyte adhesiveness, content of fibrinogen and the size, gross and net weights of invitro thrombus, thus offering some hemorrheological clues and materials for exploring the mechanism of the therapy.

*Materials and methods*

(a) Dogs of both sexes were collected from rural areas; body weight ranged between 14 and 20 kg.

(b) Equipment:

—WTP-A type Chinese-made apparatus for measuring thrombosis and adhesion of platelets.

—WTP BI type Chinese-made adjustable barostatic capillary viscosimetre.

(c) Method: Five dogs were anesthetized with 1 ml/kg 3% Na-pentobarbital intraperitoneally. Blood specimens were obtained via the great saphenous vein 30 minutes before and 30 minutes after acupressure manipulation.

(1) Measurement of the length, gross weight and net weight of invitro thrombus.

The blood specimen was anticoagulated with 3.8% Na citrate in a ratio of 1:9. Add 0.2 ml of 1.25% Cac 12 to each ml of anticoagulant blood and leave it in a silicified plastic test tube. Let the tube whirl on the turntable of the invitro thrombometre for 10 minutes. Pour out the thrombus from the tube onto a filter paper. Pick up one end of the thrombus with a tweezer and let it hang naturally. Put it on a pre-weighed filter paper to measure its length. Weigh the thrombus with the filter paper. The gross weight of the thrombus is thus obtained by deducting the weight of the filter paper. Then dry the wet thrombus and filter paper in the hemostat oven at 64 °C for 20 minutes. The net weight of the dried thrombus is obtained by deducting the weight of the filter paper.

(2) Measurement of plasma viscosity.

Three ml. of anticoagulant blood was centrifuged at a speed of 3000 cycles/min. for 8 minutes. The plasma was taken out and placed in a silicified test tube and pre-heated in a pre-heating pool of plasmal viscosimetre set at 37 °C. First, the time for 1 ml. of distilled water to pass through the capillary was measured. Then the time taken by 1 ml. of pre-heated plasma was measured and this step was repeated. The figure obtained from the third measurement was used for calculation.

The plasmal viscosity of all the specimen was measured in the same way.

$$\eta \text{ specimen} = \frac{t \text{ specimen}}{t \text{ distilled water}} \times 0.6915 \text{ unit: mPa·S}$$

Notice: $\eta$ = Mask of blood viscosity

(3) Measurement of content of fibrinogen.

Pour 10 mm. of the plasma obtained from the anticoagulant blood into a silicified test tube. The tube was put into a thermostat at 56 °C and heated for 10 minutes. The plasma was then centrifuged at 3000 cycles/min. for 10 minutes. The readings of fibrinogen on the scale of the tube were taken and the content of fibrinogen (mg%) was calculated.

(4) Measurement of erythrocyte sedimentation rate (ESR).

The ESR (mm/hr.) was measured by placing the anticoagulant blood in the test tube up to the 10 ml. mark and leaving it on the stand for 1 hour at room temperature.

(5) Measurement of red cell volume.

The percentage figure was obtained by centrifuging the tube for ESR at 3000 cycles/min. for 1/2 hour.

(6) Measurement of the rate of platelet adhesiveness.

Half a ml. of 3.13% Na-citrate was mixed with 4.5 ml. of whole blood. After anticoagulation, 1.5 ml. was drawn and placed in a small silicified glass ball which was rotated on a turntable for 15 minutes at 3 cycles/sec. 1 ml. of anticoagulant blood (before adhesion) and another 1 ml. from the glass ball (after adhesion) were each mixed with 19 ml. of 3.13% Na-citrate and left to stand for 2 hours. 10 ml. of supernatant was dropped into a cell counter and left to stand for 15 minutes. The platelets were counted and the rate of adhesion worked out according to the following formula:

Rate of platelet adhesiveness% = Difference between platelet count before and after contact/Platelet count before contact × 100

(7) Measurement of whole blood viscosity.

The process of anticoagulation, the measurement of the time required for whole blood 1 ml. to pass through the capillary, and the determination of whole blood viscosity all followed the same methods and formula used for working out plasma viscosity as stated in (2) in the above.

*Result*

The animal experiment was repeated twice, and the results were compared and verified as follows:

(a) Effect of acupressure manipulation on the length, gross weight and net weight of the thrombus invitro.

**Table 31**

| A single acupressure manipulation | Number of dogs tested | Length of thrombus (cm) | p value | Gross weight of vet thrombus (g) | p value | Net weight of dried thrombus (g) | p value |
|---|---|---|---|---|---|---|---|
| Before | | 2.125 ± 0.9125 | | 0.1377 ± 0.0553 | | 0.0959 ± 0.0107 | |
| | 4 | | ‹ 0.02 | | ›0.05 | | › 0.05 |
| After | | 0.55 ± 0.4123 | | 0.0327 ± 0.0107 | | 0.0376 ± 0.0423 | |

The result showed that the length of the thrombus after manipulation is markedly shortened, the statistical difference being very significant. There was an obvious tendency for the gross and net weights of the thrombus to decrease. (See Fig. 96)

(b) Effect of acupressure manipulation on whole blood viscosity and plasma viscosity. (See Fig. 97)

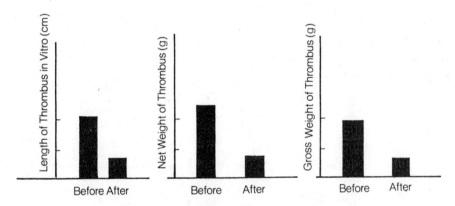

**Fig. 96    Effect of acupressure manipulation on the in vitro length, gross and net weights of thrombus in dogs before and after a single manipulation**

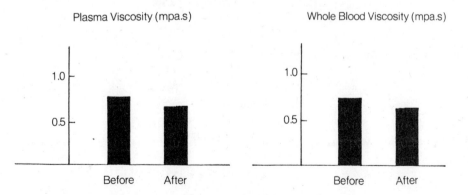

**Fig. 97    Effect of acupressure manipulation on whole blood and plasma viscosities in dogs before and after manipulation**

**Table 32**

| Lot number | Manipulation | Number of dogs tested | Plasmal viscosity (mpa.s) | p value | Viscosity of whole blood (mp.s) | p value |
|---|---|---|---|---|---|---|
| First lot | Before | 5 | 0.70214 ± 0.004 | ‹ 0.01 | 0.71642 ± 0.006 | ‹ 0.02 |
|  | After |  | 0.69352 ± 0.002 |  | 0.7078 ± 0.0039 |  |
| Second lot | Before | 5 | 0.70106 ± 0.004 | ‹ 0.05 | 0.70854 ± 0.0018 | ‹ 0.001 |
|  | After |  | 0.69528 ± 0.00176 |  | 0.69796 ± 0.00148 |  |

(c) Effect of acupressure manipulation on the rate of adhesiveness of platelets. (See Fig. 98)

Results showed a remarkable change in the adhesiveness of platelets before and after manipulation. There was an obvious decrease in the adhesiveness of platelets after manipulation.

**Table 33**

| Lot number | Manipulation | Number of dogs tested | Rate of platelet adhesiveness (%) | p value |
|---|---|---|---|---|
| First lot | Before | 5 | 41.8 ± 2.168 | › 0.05 |
|  | After |  | 31.4 ± 9.762 |  |
| Second lot | Before | 5 | 46.12 ± 10.854 | ‹ 0.01 |
|  | After |  | 20.12 ± 9.1906 |  |

(d) Effect of acupressure manipulation on the content of fibrinogen. (See Fig. 99)

**Table 34**

| Lot number | Manipulation | Number of dogs tested | Content of fibrinogen (mg%) | p value |
|---|---|---|---|---|
| First lot | Before | 5 | 252 ± 26.83 | ‹ 0.01 |
|  | After |  | 180 ± 42.43 |  |
| Second lot | Before | 5 | 354 ± 124.0161 | › 0.05 |
|  | After |  | 220 ± 26.8323 |  |

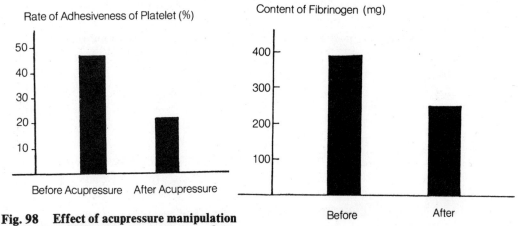

**Fig. 98    Effect of acupressure manipulation on the rate of adhesiveness of platelet in dogs**

**Fig. 99    Effect of acupressure manipulation on the content of fibrinogen in dogs**

Results showed that the content of fibrinogen after manipulation was markedly lower than that before manipulation.

(e) Effect of acupressure manipulation on the ESR and blood cell volume.

**Table 35**

| Lot number | Manipulation | Number of dogs tested | EST (mm.hr.) | P value | Blood cell volume | p value |
|---|---|---|---|---|---|---|
| First lot | Before | | $33.8 \pm 22.38$ | | $28 \pm 8.06$ | |
| | | 5 | | $< 0.05$ | | $> 0.05$ |
| | After | | $30.8 \pm 17.796$ | | $28.8 \pm 1.30$ | |
| Second lot | Before | | $7.8 \pm 9.859$ | | $34.2 \pm 3.5637$ | |
| | | 5 | | $> 0.05$ | | $> 0.05$ |
| | After | | $7.2 \pm 12.755$ | | $37 \pm 5.2915$ | |

Results showed that there was a tendency of ESR and blood cell volume to decrease after acupressure manipulation.

*Discussion*

According to traditional Chinese medicine, sequelae of cerebral birth injury and other traumatic paralyses are caused by the blocking of meridians and the stagnation of blood and vital energy as a result of external injuries that lead to extremity numbness and inability to move and acupressure therapy "removes obstruction in the flow of vital energy by pressing the meridians and treats stagnation by massaging the lump," so that the flow of vital energy in the meridians is restored, harmony between energy and blood is achieved, blood circulation is activated and stagnant blood is cleared. The "Tentative Standard for the Diagnosis of Blood Stagnation," adopted in 1982 at the First National Symposium on Activating Blood-Circulation and Dissipating

Blood-Stagnation, sponsored by the Chinese Association of Integrated Traditional and Western Medicine has reaffirmed that blood stagnation is a cause of extremity numbness and hemiparalysis, and is therefore an objective indicator for the diagnosis of blood stagnation syndrome. The symposium also agreed that in case of blood stagnation, hemorrheological changes are manifestations of changes in the quality and constitution of blood, as it turns into a thick, viscous and highly coagulated state.

Lab experimentation with dogs showed that after acupressure manipulation, there was a marked decrease in fibrinogen content and the rate of platelet adhesiveness, a shortening of the length of invitro thrombus, a tendency for the gross and net weights of the thrombus to decrease and a decrease in ESR and blood cell hematocrit. All this may well be accompanied by simultaneous changes in the thick, viscous and highly coagulated state of the stagnated blood. This offers objective evidence of acupressure's mechanism of activating blood circulation and dissipating blood stagnancy.

Modern medical science holds that sequelae of cerebral birth injury are caused mainly by protracted or difficult labour, resulting in prolongation of the delivery process or traumatic injuries, which, in turn, cause cerebral ischemia, disturbance of microcirculation, encephaledema and cellular anoxia. These disorders degenerate or necrose the tissues and cells in the cerebral motor and sensory areas, causing extremity numbness and motor disturbance. The effect of acupressure therapy on the thrombus, the whole blood and plasma viscosity, the adhesiveness of platelets, fibrinogen and ECR and blood cell volume, as stated in the above, demonstrates that it is beneficial in activating the tissue metabolism in the tissue, restoring the function of neurocytes in the area of the brain lesion, activating static neurocytes and improving the functions of the affected limbs in general.

Since animal models of sequelae of cerebral birth injury were not available for experimentation, normal animals were used to observe the hemorrheological changes before and after acupressure treatment a factor that should be taken into consideration in the evaluation of the results.

### 6. Effect of acupressure manipulation on the neurotransmitter in dog's blood

Through observation of the SEP, it has been found that after receiving acupressure therapy, the latent period was shortened, i.e., the velocity of neural transmission was accelerated. Moreover, by observing the microcirculation in both patients and experimental animals, it has been found that after acupressure therapy, both the calibers of the capillaries and the blood flow increased, indicating the direct action of acupressure therapy on the nerves and blood vessels of the organism. In order to probe into the mechanism, experimental dogs were used so as to observe the changes in the neurotransmitter in blood, including nor-adrenalin (NE), adrenalin (E), 5-hydroxytryptamine (5HT), 5-hydroxyindole acetic acid (5-HIAA), dopamine (DA) and cholinesterase activity, both before and after acupressure treatment.

*Materials and methods*

(a) Main reagents:

(1) Di-noradrenalin bi-tartrate

(2) Dopamine-hydrochlorate

(3) 5-hydroxytryptamine creatinine hydrochloric acid

(4) 5-hydroxyindole acetic acid

(5) Adrenalin

(6) Acetylcholine

(7) N-butyl alcohol

(8) N-heptane

(9) O-phthalate adehyde

(10) Sodium periodate

(11) Sodium molybdate

(12) Potassium arsenate

(13) Hydroxylamine hydrochlorate

(14) Ferric chloride

(b) Instruments

(1) HITACHI 850-fluorescent spectrophotometre.

(2) BECKMAN Du-8B spectrophotometre.

(c) Animals and mode of drawing blood specimens.

Domestic dogs weighing 14-20 kg each from villages were administered with helminthics and given quarantine inspection for 2 weeks. After intraperitoneal anesthesia with 3% Na-pentobarbilol in 1 ml./kg dosage, blood was drawn through the great saphenous vein. Imitated clinical acupressure manipulation lasting 20 minutes was given, following which blood specimens were drawn immediately. A second lot was drawn 40 minutes later. There were altogether 3 lots of blood specimens.

(d) Method of measurement

Each blood specimen was divided into 3 portions:

(1) Mix 0.1 ml. blood with 0.5 ml. saline and shake. De-proteinize the specimen by adding 10% and 3% tro-chloroacetic acid. The supernatant fluid was measured for adrenaline by the adsorption method.

(2) 0.5 ml. of blood with K-oxalate was used for measuring whole blood cholinesterase by the colorimetric method.

(3) Take plasma from 1.5 cc of whole blood with heparin. Add 0.6 N trichloroacetic acid to de-prateinize the specimen, from which the supernatant fluid has been diluted four times. Extract with ortho-butyl alcohol and measure water phase for its 5-hydroxyindole acetic acid content, while the organic phase is extracted with 5-hydroxytryptamine, nor-adrenalin and dopamine into 0.1 N Hcl for further measurement. 5-HT, 5-HIAA and 0-phthalate aldehyde underwent condensation reaction and were examined separately with 475/560 and 480/550 mu wave length in the HITACHI 850 fluorescent spectrophotographer. After being oxygenated with iodine, specimen measurement was made by 370/430 and 373/420 mu wave length for NE and DA respectively with the above instrument. The ng/ml. value was obtained by calculating the integral value against the standard curve.

*Results*

(a) Changes in blood 5-HT, 5-HIAA, NE and DA.

As shown in Table 36, after manipulation, the blood showed a decrease in varying degrees in the catecholamine substances of NE and DA. Though the statistical difference was not significant, the level of the content dropped with the lapse of time.

This showed that the changes might follow a pattern. (See Fig. 100) The 5-HIAA and 5-HT values all increased after acupressure manipulation, the former showed significant statistical difference (P < 0.01). (See Fig. 101)

**Table 36　Changes in Monoamine Substances in Dogs' Blood Before and After Acupressure Manipulation**

| Substances measured | Number of dogs tested | Results X ± SD (ng/ml.) | | |
|---|---|---|---|---|
| | | Before manipulation | Immediately after manipulation | 40 minutes after manipulation |
| NE | 8 | 79.77 ± 6.83 | 75.85 ± 5.46 | 72.71 ± 3.36* |
| DA | 8 | 658.05 ± 86.2 | 601.94 ± 67.2 | 580.46 ± 26.43 |
| 5-HIAA | 9 | 6.07 ± 2.22 | 7.25 ± 2.67 | 7.46 ± 2.89** |
| 5-HT | 8 | 8.84 ± 3.0 | 12.6 ± 11.9 | 16.46 ± 16.46 |

*Compared with pre-manipulation value, P = 0.05.
**Compared with pre-manipulation value, P < 0.01.

**Table 37　Changes in Blood 5-HT/NE, 5-HT/DA Before and After Acupressure Manipulation in Dogs**

| Item | Ratio on the basis of different time phases | | |
|---|---|---|---|
| | Before manipulation | Immediately after manipulation | 40 minutes after manipulation |
| 5-HT/NE | 0.1108 | 0.1661 | 0.2808 |
| 5-HT/DA | 0.0134 | 0.0209 | 0.0284 |

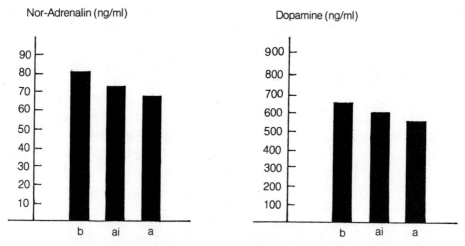

**Fig. 100　Changes in monoamine substances in dogs' blood Ne, Da before and after acupressure manipulation**

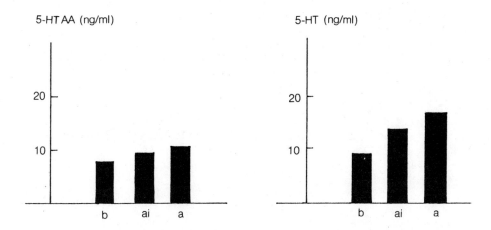

**Fig. 101    Changes in monoamine substances in dogs' blood 5-HT AA,
5-HT before and after acupressure manipulation**

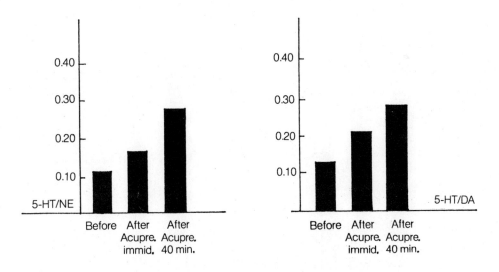

**Fig. 102    Rate of 5-HT/NE and 5-HT/DA**

It is obvious from the table after acupressure that the ratios of the 2 items continued to increase with the lapse of time, which explains the pattern of decrease in catecholamine substances and increase in 5-hydroxytryptamine substances after acupressure. (See Fig. 102)

(b) Changes in blood adrenalin.

**Table 38    Changes in Blood Adrenalin in Dogs Before and After Acupressure Manipulation**

| Time phase measured | Result X ± SD (ng/ml.) |
| --- | --- |
| Before manipulation | 11.33 ± 2.44 |
| Immediately after manipulation | 12.67 ± .2.09 |
| 40 minutes after manipulation | 12.19 ± 1.14 |

No obvious changes are seen from the above table in the blood adrenalin content before and after acupressure manipulation.

(c) Changes in blood cholinesterase activity.

**Table 39    Changes in Blood Cholinesterase Activity Before and After
Acupressure Manipulation in Dogs**

| Time phase measured | Results X ± SD (ng/ml.) |
| --- | --- |
| Before manipulation | 28.91 ± 11.01 |
| Immediately after manipulation | 18.15 ± 7.38* |
| 40 minutes after manipulation | 23.29 ± 8.80 |

*As compared with that before manipulation, P < 0.05.

The above table 39 shows that after receiving acupressure manipulation, the activity of blood cholinesterase markedly decreased. After 40 minutes, the corresponding figures rose. (See Fig. 103)

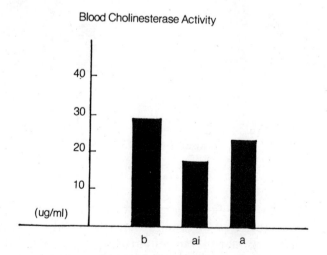

**Fig. 103    Changes of blood cholinesterase activity
before and after acupressure manipulation in dogs**

*Analysis of the results*

(a) The experiments provided positive evidence regarding the clinical effect of acupressure therapy, as demonstrated in the improvement of microcirculation; the decrease of hyper-viscosity, hyper-adhesiveness and hyper-coagulating tendency of the blood; as well as the shortening of the latent period of somatosensory evoked potential. Thus, it is apparent that there is a material basis for claiming the efficacy of acupressure treatment, at least there is evidence that the therapy is related to the neuro-transmitter in the body. As the levels of NE and DA in the peripheral circulation decrease, resulting in vaso-dilalation and increase of blood flow, the nutritional supply of the body and the cerebrum are improved, which is beneficial to the recovery of tissue cells in the lesions. Of course, the physiological actions of NE and DA within the brain and in the peripheral circulatory system cannot be interpreted simply by excitation and inhibition. Nevertheless the satisfactory clinical results of acupressure therapy might be related to the action of NE and DA on the motor function of the body, pituitory hormone secretion, and the regulation of the cardiovascular system and psychoneural activities. Increase in the contents of 5-HT, 5-HIAA in the blood after acupressure manipulation is again related to psychoneural hormone regulation. Lowering of cholinesterase activity denotes less destruction of acetylcholine, loading to its relative increase in content. As a result, it is beneficial to the excitation of muscle fibers and the strengthening of muscle contraction, which brings various physiological activities up to their normal level. It has been reported that acetylcholine exerts a remarkable influence on the near and distant memory of the brain. The recovery of motor function, improved intelligence and recovery from aphasia after acupressure therapy might be in some way related to the change in the neurotransmitter.

(b) Whether or not the change in the neurotransmitter is specifically one evoked by acupressure therapy is still under investigation. The results of the experimentation are similar to those obtained by the researchers in the Nanjing College of Traditional Chinese Medicine, who treated acute injury of the soft tissues by massage. They revealed that after massage treatment, blood NE and DA decreased markedly, while 5-HT and 5-HIAA either remained basically unchanged or showed a tendency to increase. It may be concluded that similar changes would occur when manipulating the body by means of pressing, massaging or percussing techniques.

(c) It is presumed that if the experimentation was conducted on animal models suffering from sequelae of cerebral birth injury, and the results could be examined with the animals restored to their senses, the changes before and after acupressure would be more clearly reflected. The very low level of 5-HT and 5-HIAA in the experimentation under study might be the result of anesthetization of these animals.

Conclusion

Derived from Chinese martial arts, acupressure therapy is a valuable legacy of traditional Chinese medicine. Acupressure techniques in Chinese martial art have a history of some two thousand years, and are well-known amongst the Chinese people. The earliest written record, however, was found in the *History of the Ming Dynasty* (1368-1644), and was incomplete. There was no report on its therapeutic value. After the founding of the People's Republic, the technique of acupressure therapy was clinically applied with satisfactory results. In the 1960s, the therapy was used for the treatment of infantile paralysis; while in the 80s, its clinical application was extended to a large number of other patients. Scientific research followed and yielded satisfactory results.

Why can acupressure therapy cure many diseases? According to traditional Chinese medical theory, vital energy and blood are the essence of human life. When they co-exist in a state or condition of harmony, the life-force will be vital and strong; whilst their disharmony on the other hand can eventually result in an end to life itself. Acupressure therapy treats patients by applying digital force to the vital acupoints, with treatment varying according to the individual's constitution, age and general condition. Integrated with the principles of Yin and Yang, tonification and purgation, acupressure techniques direct vital energy and blood flow towards the sites of lesion, resulting in the dredging of the meridians, relief of spasm and improvement or complete recovery of body functions.

Not content with clinical results, doctors and researchers have probed into the mechanism of the therapy by means of the study of sequelae of cerebral birth injury. Since the lesions are in the brain, the studies began with cerebral blood circulation. Taking the TCM approach of "activating blood circulation and dissipating blood stagnation" as their point of departure, studies were made on the hemodynamics of cerebral blood flow. Using gamma photography to record the changes in dogs' cerebral microcirculation, which is impossible to perform invivo in humans, the following findings were made: acceleration of cerebral blood flow, increase of blood perfusion and improvement in cerebral blood circulation—all this vindicating the TCM principle of "activating blood circulation and dissipating blood stagnation." Besides, examination of microcirculation in patients' fingernail-fold and measurement of dogs' hemorrheology revealed results that tallied with the same principles. It can thus be claimed that acupressure therapy improves not only peripheral blood circulation, but also cerebral blood circulation. It is commonly known that affection of neurocytes at the lesion of the central nervous system is irreversible. However, the portion around the lesion and a large number of normal neurocytes remain in a state of rest. By stimulating and increasing the cerebral blood circulation, acupressure therapy may reactivate the resting cells, thereby restoring functional activities and accelerating the convalescence of the affected limbs. Hence, the clinical effect.

Experiments on the blood neurotransmitter have also revealed results which support the above hypothesis of "activating blood circulation and dissipating blood stagnation." Somatosensory evoked potential also proved that the therapy improve the conducting function of the nervous system.

The following diagrams encapsulate the mechanism of acupressure therapy:

Acknowledgement

Many thanks go to Yun Shizhong, Wu Xiabo, Lu Zhufeng, Bai Yuxi, Bai Guoqing, Han Fengyue, Yang Meixiang, Chen Yanping and Dong Xujing for their contributions to the clinical and laboratory research work that has made this study possible.

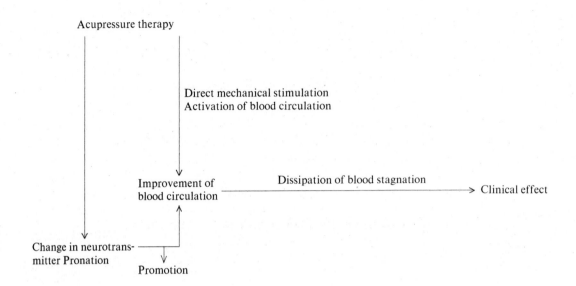

# Bibliography

1. Jia Lihui, et al, *Pointing Therapy*, Shandong Science and Technology Press, 1986.

2. Cheng Xinnong, *Chinese Acupuncture and Moxibustion*, Foreign Languages Press, Beijing, 1987.

3. Wang Zhongcheng, *Neurosurgery*, People's Health Publishing House, 1978.

4. Feng Tianyou, *Treatment of Soft Tissue Injury by Integrated Methods of Traditional Chinese and Western Medicine*, People's Health Publishing House, 1977.

5. Cheng Zhengguang, *Teaching Material of Soft Tissue Injury*, the Institute of Orthopaedics and Traumatology, China Academy of Traditional Chinese Medicine, 1984.

6. Liu Lei, et al, *Principle of Electroneuromyography*, Science Press, 1983.

7. Starr, I., et al, *Circulation*, v. 9, p. 468, May 1954.

8. Xie Shaowen: *Progress in Experimental Cellulal Immunology*, Volume I, Institute of Medical Information, Chinese Academy of Medical Sciences, 1980.

9. Wang Zhaopu, et al, "Preliminary Observation of 150 Cases of Sequelae of Cerebral Birth Injury in Infants Treated by Acupressure Therapy," *Journal of Traditional Chinese Medicine*, v. 27, p. 38, June 1986.

10. Beijing College of Traditional Chinese Medicine, *Teaching Material on Acupuncture and Moxibustion*, May 1975.

11. Wang Yici, et al, "Study on Cortical Evoked Potential in Incomplete Cranial Paralysis due to Asphyxiation in Newborn Infants," *Journal of Apoplexy and Nervous Disease*, v. 3, p. 146, March 1986.

12. Xiu Ruijuan, et al, *Disturbance of Microcirculation and Its Related Diseases*, Henan Science and Technology Press, 1985.

13. Zhao Huiyang, et al, "Methods in Encephalo-Scanning," *Nuclear Medicine*, Shanghai Science and Technology Press, 1981.

14. Graham, D.I., "Pathology of Cerebral Ischemia and Methods of Treatment," *Foreign Medicine, Volume on Anesthesia and Resurrenction*, p. 54, 1981.

15. Beijing Children's Hospital, *Encephalo-Paralysis in Applied Pediatrics*.

16. Deng Xixian, "Progress in Research on Circulation Physiology," *Year Book of Chinese Medical Sciences*, p. 122, 1984.

17. Yuan Shenyuan, et al, "Automatic Measuring System for Velocity of Capillary Blood Flow and Its Application," *Chinese Medical Journal,* v. 62, August 1982.

18. Tian Niu, Shan Yi, "Velocity of Blood-Flow of Microcirculation of the Nail-Fold," *Handbook of Clinical Examination on Nail Fold Microcirculation*, p. 49, 1987.

19. Jin Huiming, "Progress in the Study of Microcirculation," *Chinese Medical Journal*, v. 62, p. 497, August 1982.

20. Beijing College of Traditional Chinese Medicine, *Fundamentals of Traditional*

*Chinese Medicine,* March 1974.

21. Mao Tengmin, et al, "Exploration into Pathology of Models of Blood Stagnation," *Bulletin of Beijing Medical College,* v. 17, p. 252, April 1985.

22. Proposal made at the First National Symposium on Activating Blood Circulation and Dissipating Blood Stagnation, Sponsored by the Chinese Association of Integrated Traditional and Western Medicine, "Tentative Standards for Diagnosis of Blood Stagnation Syndrome," *Journal of Integrated Traditional and Chinese Medicine,* v. 3, *inside cover,* March 1983.

23. Compiled by Chen Guiting, "Minutes of National Symposium on Modern Research in the Theory of Traditional Chinese Medicine (2)," "Discussion on Modern Research in the Theory of Traditional Chinese Medicine," August 1987.

24. Zhao Jiahong, "On the Relation Between Qi-Blood (Vital Energy-Blood) and Injury," *Papers Presented to the National Symposium on Orthopedics and Traumatology in Traditional Chinese Medicine,* p. 5, 1983.

25. Xiao Junfeng, "Application of the Treatment Principle for Activating Blood Circulation and Dissipating Blood Stagnation in Orthopedic-Traumatic Diseases," *Papers Presented to the National Symposium on Orthopedic & Traumatology in TCM,* 1983.

26. MAT A v. 5, p. 26, 1961.

27. *Clinical Biochemical Examination* (Vol. 1), Shanghai Science & Technology Press, 1979.

28. Department of Biochemistry, Institute of Acu-moxibustion, Chinese Academy of Traditional Chinese Medicine, *Reference to TCM,* 1979.

29. Liu Zhicheng, et al, *Chinese Journal of Rehabilitation Medicine,* v. 1, p. 8, March 1986.

30. Beijing Medical College, *Biochemistry,* p. 461, 1978.

**图书在版编目(CIP)数据**

中国点穴疗法:英文/王肇普著;彭瑞复审校 .—北京:外文出版社,1999
ISBN 7－119－02056－0

Ⅰ.中… Ⅱ.①王… ②彭… Ⅲ.穴位按压疗法－英文 Ⅳ.R244.1

中国版本图书馆 CIP 数据核字 (97) 第 12264 号

责任编辑　胡开敏
封面设计　王　志

外文出版社网址:
　http://www.flp.com.cn
外文出版社电子信箱:
　info@flp.com.cn
　sales@flp.com.cn

**中国点穴疗法**

王肇普　著

\*

ⓒ外文出版社
外文出版社出版
(中国北京百万庄大街 24 号)
邮政编码 100037
北京外文印刷厂印刷
中国国际图书贸易总公司发行
(中国北京车公庄西路 35 号)
北京邮政信箱第 399 号　邮政编码 100044
1999 年(16 开)第 1 版
1999 年第 1 版第 1 次印刷
(英)
ISBN 7－119－02056－0/R·154(外)
07400
14－E－3201S